MCQs in
Physical Medicine and
Rehabilitation

MCQs in Physical Medicine and Rehabilitation

Previously known as MCQs in Rehabilitation Medicine

Second Edition

S Sunder MBBS MD (PMR)
Consultant
Department of Physical Medicine and Rehabilitation
JOGO Health Inc, USA

Co-author
Jimi Jose MBBS MD DNB (PMR)
Assistant Professor
Department of Physical Medicine and Rehabilitation
Pushpagiri Medical College
Thiruvalla, Kerala, India

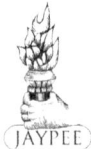

JAYPEE BROTHERS MEDICAL PUBLISHERS
The Health Sciences Publisher
New Delhi | London

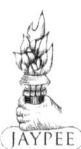 **Jaypee Brothers Medical Publishers (P) Ltd**

Headquarters
Jaypee Brothers Medical Publishers (P) Ltd
EMCA House
23/23-B, Ansari Road, Daryaganj
New Delhi - 110 002, India
Landline: +91-11-23272143, +91-11-23272703
+91-11-23282021, +91-11-23245672
Email: jaypee@jaypeebrothers.com

Corporate Office
Jaypee Brothers Medical Publishers (P) Ltd
4838/24, Ansari Road, Daryaganj
New Delhi 110 002, India
Phone: +91-11-43574357
Fax: +91-11-43574314
Email: jaypee@jaypeebrothers.com
Website: www.jaypeebrothers.com

Overseas office
J.P. Medical Ltd
83 Victoria Street, London
SW1H 0HW (UK)
Phone: +44 20 3170 8910
Fax: +44 (0)20 3008 6180
Email: info@jpmedpub.com

Website: www.jaypeedigital.com

© 2022, Jaypee Brothers Medical Publishers

The views and opinions expressed in this book are solely those of the original contributor(s)/author(s) and do not necessarily represent those of editor(s) of the book.

All rights reserved. No part of this publication may be reproduced, stored or transmitted in any form or by any means, electronic, mechanical, photocopying, recording or otherwise, without the prior permission in writing of the publishers.

All brand names and product names used in this book are trade names, service marks, trademarks or registered trademarks of their respective owners. The publisher is not associated with any product or vendor mentioned in this book.

Medical knowledge and practice change constantly. This book is designed to provide accurate, authoritative information about the subject matter in question. However, readers are advised to check the most current information available on procedures included and check information from the manufacturer of each product to be administered, to verify the recommended dose, formula, method and duration of administration, adverse effects and contraindications. It is the responsibility of the practitioner to take all appropriate safety precautions. Neither the publisher nor the author(s)/editor(s) assume any liability for any injury and/or damage to persons or property arising from or related to use of material in this book.

This book is sold on the understanding that the publisher is not engaged in providing professional medical services. If such advice or services are required, the services of a competent medical professional should be sought.

Every effort has been made where necessary to contact holders of copyright to obtain permission to reproduce copyright material. If any have been inadvertently overlooked, the publisher will be pleased to make the necessary arrangements at the first opportunity.

Inquiries for bulk sales may be solicited at: jaypee@jaypeebrothers.com

MCQs in Physical Medicine and Rehabilitation

First Edition: 2005
Second Edition: **2022**
ISBN 978-93-5465-489-3

Preface to the Second Edition

The fourth edition of the popular *Textbook of Rehabilitation* came out in November 2019, around the time the subject of Physical Medicine and Rehabilitation (PM&R) was being included in the medical curriculum. PM&R, representing one of the important phases of medical care, and which focuses on quality of life, is thus becoming an integral part of the study of medicine. One of the many ways a medical student is tested is through MCQs or multiple choice questions. Many universities have included MCQs in their examination systems and this handbook of multiple choice questions, broadly based on the chapters in the textbook would help in such a situation.

With the advent of technology and information sharing, medical knowledge has been expanding exponentially. The rapid advancements in medical information are mirrored by an estimated 2 million scientific research articles published every year, in some 25,000 to 30,000 medical journals. The doubling time of added medical information was an estimated 50 years back in 1950, accelerated to 7 years in 1980, and is estimated to be 73 days by 2020. The questions in this book are therefore based on information available to us from various sources but which is always subject to dynamic change. We have also tried to take into consideration regional differences to determine the relevance of these MCQs.

We have tried to include as many questions as possible with a focus on rehabilitation, but naturally there will be considerable overlap with the specialties of neurology, orthopedics or rheumatology. Wherever there are answers which arguably may be correct, the correct answer is the ***nearest one*** to whatever goes by current medical practice and evidence-based knowledge at the time of publication. Also, it is possible that some questions may be relevant in another chapter, for example, a question in the chapter on Therapeutic Exercises and Techniques could very well fit in the chapter on Orthopedics and Sports Rehabilitation. Questions in any chapter have to be taken as far as possible as relevant to that chapter. I am sure that this book will be of great use to the medical community at large, and also to any professional interested in the field of rehabilitation.

This book's co-author, Dr Jimi Jose has joined me in preparing several of the questions and answers and both of us have served as sounding boards for each other while discussing the right answers. He has contributed immensely to the content, including some chapters. I wish to thank Ms Ranjini Narayan, for her inputs in the chapter on Management of Behavioral and Learning Problems.

S Sunder

Preface to the First Edition

Close on the heels of the popular *Textbook of Rehabilitation*, comes this little handbook of multiple choice questions in the same subject. Many universities have included MCQs in their examination systems and rehabilitation is no exception.

I am sure that this book will be of great use not only to students of physiotherapy and occupational therapy but also to the medical community at large.

I wish to acknowledge the help rendered to me by Ms Anagha and Ms Narayanee, in bringing out this book.

S Sunder

Contents

Section I: General Principles

1. Introduction to Rehabilitation Medicine 3
2. The Rehabilitation Team 7
3. Sociolegal Aspects of Rehabilitation 11
4. Architectural Barriers 15
5. Activities of Daily Living 19

Section II: Therapeutic Management

6. Therapeutic Exercises and Techniques 25
7. Clinical Examination 30
8. Gait 34
9. Hand Function and Occupational Therapy 38
10. Management of Communication Impairment 42
11. Management of Behavioral and Learning Problems 46
12. Orthotics 52
13. Prosthetics 58
14. Mobility Aids 63
15. Vocational Rehabilitation 67
16. Pain and Musculoskeletal Disorders 71
17. Surgery in Rehabilitation 75
18. Physical Agents 79

Section III: Management of Special Populations

19. Hereditary and Congenital Problems 87
20. Ergonomics 91

Section IV: Medical Conditions Needing Rehabilitation

21. Burns 97

22. Brain Injury and Stroke 101
23. Lower Motor Neuron Lesions 106
24. Pediatric Rehabilitation and Cerebral Palsy 111
25. Orthopedics and Sports Rehabilitation 115
26. Diseases of the Muscle 121
27. Spinal Cord Injury 125
28. Movement Disorders 131
29. Cardiopulmonary Rehabilitation 135
30. Vascular and Hematological Conditions 139
31. Arthritis 143

SECTION I: General Principles

SECTION OUTLINE

1. Introduction to Rehabilitation Medicine
2. The Rehabilitation Team
3. Sociolegal Aspects of Rehabilitation
4. Architectural Barriers
5. Activities of Daily Living

CHAPTER 1

Introduction to Rehabilitation Medicine

1. Benefits of mobility in a bed-ridden patient include the following, *except*:
   A. Prevention of disuse atrophy
   B. Prevention of contractures
   C. Prevention of pressure sores
   D. Prevention of stroke
2. Which of these is a handicap for a person with disability?
   A. Laryngectomy
   B. Anisognosia
   C. Lack of vocational training
   D. Difficulty in using the right upper limb in a right-handed individual
3. Which of these is a disability?
   A. Hemimelia
   B. Spina bifida
   C. Congenital Talipes equinovarus
   D. Partial hearing loss in the right ear
4. The most common handicap according to the 2011 census in India is:
   A. Visual handicap
   B. Hearing impairment
   C. Mental handicap
   D. Locomotor handicap

1. D   2. C   3. D   4. D

Section I: General Principles

5. Examples of impairment secondary to a primary disability include all the following, *except*:
   A. Pressure sores
   B. Stroke
   C. Equinus in poliomyelitis
   D. Heterotopic ossification
6. Any loss or abnormality of psychological, physiological or anatomical nature is known as:
   A. Disability
   B. Impairment
   C. Deformity
   D. Handicap
7. The incidence of disability in the Indian census 2011 is estimated to be around:
   A. 3.5%
   B. 2.2%
   C. 1%
   D. 7.5%
8. Rehabilitation is the phase of medical care conjointly with or immediately after the following, *except*:
   A. Preventive phase
   B. Acute phase
   C. Curative phase
   D. Surgical phase
9. Post-traumatic amputation of a finger is:
   A. Impairment
   B. Disability
   C. Handicap
   D. Secondary disability
10. A child with disability should:
    A. Be protected from society
    B. Not be allowed to play with other children who are similarly disabled
    C. Not be allowed to go to school at a very early age
    D. Be encouraged for social interaction
11. Rehabilitation of a disease or condition comes under:
    A. Primary prevention
    B. Secondary prevention
    C. Tertiary prevention
    D. Quarternary prevention

5. B   6. B   7. B   8. A   9. A   10. D
11. C

Chapter 1: Introduction to Rehabilitation Medicine

12. What the person with disability can do or perform at the time of being assessed is called:
    A. Psychiatric diagnosis
    B. Functional diagnosis
    C. ADL function
    D. Physiological diagnosis
13. The inability of the person to perform an activity in the manner within the range considered as normal is:
    A. Impairment   B. Handicap
    C. Disability   D. Deformity
14. All of the following statements are correct, *except*:
    A. Impairment leads to disability
    B. All impairments lead to disability
    C. Relationship between impairment and disability is bidirectional
    D. Disability leads to handicap
15. One of the following is not an impairment
    A. Neuropraxia   B. Neurotmesis
    C. Claw hand   D. Axonotmesis
16. Children with cerebral palsy may suffer from:
    A. Locomotor disability
    B. Hearing disability
    C. Mental impairment
    D. All of the above
17. A typist who has lost a finger has a:
    A. Major impairment and minor disability
    B. Minor impairment and major disability
    C. Minor disability and major handicap
    D. Minor disability and minor handicap
18. The primary role of the medical professional in the rehabilitation team is:
    A. Vocational rehabilitation
    B. Income generation for the handicapped
    C. Disability limitation
    D. Reduction of architectural barriers

12. B   13. C   14. B   15. C   16. D   17. C
18. C

Section I: General Principles

19. A disadvantage for a given individual in his or her social context that limits or prevents the fulfilment of a role that is normal for him or her is known as:
    A. Impairment
    B. Handicap
    C. Disability
    D. Deformity
20. A patient who has suffered a stroke, and is immobile, is made to walk in an inpatient rehabilitation center. This is an example of:
    A. Reduction of handicap
    B. Disability limitation
    C. Sociovocational rehabilitation
    D. Disability evaluation
21. The goals of rehabilitation are all, *except*:
    A. Physical independence
    B. Mobility
    C. Performance of exercises
    D. Social and occupational integration
22. **Sociovocational rehabilitation:**
    A. Involves only the social worker and the vocational counsellor
    B. Does not involve medical rehabilitation personnel
    C. Starts only when medical rehabilitation is over
    D. Provides persons with disability a means to reduce handicap

19. B   20. B   21. C   22. D

CHAPTER 2

The Rehabilitation Team

1. The doctor qualified in physical and rehabilitation medicine is called:
   A. Physiatrist
   B. Psychiatrist
   C. Physician
   D. Physiotherapist
2. The following is not a member of the medical rehabilitation team:
   A. Occupational therapist
   B. Speech and language pathologist
   C. Orthotist
   D. Medical social worker
3. The person who designs a multichannel functional electrical system is:
   A. Physiatrist   B. Biomedical engineer
   C. Orthotic engineer   D. Prosthetist
4. The specialist who treats the diseases of the joints is:
   A. Neurologist   B. Oncologist
   C. Rheumatologist   D. Neurosurgeon
5. The following are members of the sociovocational team, *except*:
   A. Neurosurgeon
   B. Vocational counselor
   C. Placement officer
   D. Medical social worker

1. A   2. D   3. B   4. C   5. A

Section I: General Principles

6. The following are advantages for institutional rehabilitation, *except*:
   A. Academically oriented
   B. It is economical
   C. Research oriented
   D. Training is given

7. Patients are isolated from family in:
   A. Day care center
   B. Homes for the disabled
   C. Community based rehabilitation
   D. Outpatient rehabilitation centers

8. It is more convenient to treat patients with profound quadriplegia in all of the following models, *except*:
   A. Institutional centers
   B. Community-based rehabilitation
   C. Outpatient centers
   D. Home-based rehabilitation

9. The following are the benefits of vocal music, *except*:
   A. Controls pain and anxiety
   B. Provides a musical career
   C. Improves hearing acuity
   D. Improves speech

10. The following team member is essential in acute rehabilitative care of the patient:
    A. Horticultural therapist
    B. Social worker
    C. Skilled trainer
    D. Rehabilitation nurse

11. The _____ trains the upper limb amputee in the use of the functional upper extremity prosthesis.
    A. Orthotist
    B. Occupational therapist
    C. Physiatrist
    D. Social worker

6. B   7. B   8. C   9. C   10. D   11. B

Chapter 2: The Rehabilitation Team

12. Special schools for the mentally challenged predominantly come under the following category:
    A. Outpatient rehabilitation
    B. Inpatient center
    C. Community-based rehabilitation
    D. Day care centers
13. The following are advantages of community-based rehabilitation, *except*:
    A. Participation of patient and family
    B. Presence of complete rehabilitation team
    C. Economically viable
    D. Ideal for rural population
14. The sociovocational team reduces:
    A. Impairment
    B. Disability
    C. Handicap
    D. None of the above
15. Community-based rehabilitation is:
    A. For members of a particular community
    B. Rehabilitation in developed countries
    C. Rehabilitation care in rural set up
    D. Training the medical community in rehabilitation
16. In community-based rehabilitation, the rehabilitation specialist mainly plays a role in:
    A. Training of the local population
    B. Providing medical care
    C. Pain management
    D. Setting up orthotic and prosthetic workshops
17. The speech and language pathologist helps the patient in the area of all, *except*:
    A. Cognitive retraining
    B. Swallowing assessment
    C. Vocal reeducation
    D. Vestibular rehabilitation

12. D   13. B   14. C   15. C   16. A   17. D

Section I: General Principles

18. The definition "the art and science of directing mans participation in selected activities to restore, reinforce and enhance function or performance or decrease disability and thus, to promote health." applies to which profession:
    A. Clinical psychology
    B. Occupational therapy
    C. Special education
    D. Occupational health
19. The roles of a special educator are all, *except*:
    A. Spot the deficits in the child's functioning
    B. Working out compensatory teaching methods
    C. Helping out in the vocational training
    D. Placing the child in a suitable job
20. The physiatrist:
    A. Prescribes physical modalities of treatment
    B. Performs surgery
    C. Treats pain through interventional methods
    D. All of the above
21. Most research programs are done in:
    A. Institution-based rehabilitation
    B. Day care
    C. Camps
    D. Special schools
22. Follow up is difficult in which model of rehabilitation care:
    A. Institution-based rehabilitation
    B. Day care
    C. Camps
    D. Outpatient clinics

18. B   19. D   20. D   21. A   22. C

CHAPTER

3

Sociolegal Aspects of Rehabilitation

1. The Americans with Disability Act became law in:
   A. 1993
   B. 1795
   C. 1990
   D. July 4th 1997
2. The Rehabilitation Council of India Act [RCI Act] was passed in:
   A. 1990
   B. 1992
   C. 1994
   D. 1996
3. A locomotor disabled person is eligible for travel concession if he or she has:
   A. Not less than 50% disability
   B. Not less than 40% disability
   C. 30% disability
   D. A combined total of 60% or 30% in individual disabilities whichever is more
4. According to the RPWD Act "Dwarfism" means a medical or genetic condition resulting in an adult height of:
   A. 4 feet 11 inches or less
   B. 4 feet 8 inches or less
   C. 4 feet 10 inches or less
   D. 4 feet or less
5. The following handicap is not eligible for job reservation in central Governments for C and D posts:
   A. Locomotor
   B. Mental illness
   C. Hearing and speech
   D. None of the above

1. C   2. B   3. B   4. C   5. D

Section I: General Principles

6. **The National Institute for the Orthopedically Handicapped is in:**
   A. Bombay
   B. Bangalore
   C. Kolkata
   D. Ministry of Welfare, New Delhi

7. **The public sector company ALIMCO manufacturing aids and appliances for the disabled is headquartered at:**
   A. Kochi
   B. Chennai
   C. Kanpur
   D. Patna

8. **The Act presented in India for disabilities is:**
   A. People Disability Act (PDA)
   B. National Disability Act (NDA)
   C. People with Disability Act (PWD)
   D. None of the above

9. **One of the following statements is false:**
   A. The government gives scholarships to persons with disability
   B. The government assists organizations working for persons with disability
   C. The government assists persons with disability to purchase orthoses
   D. The government provides travel concession for all persons with disability in the Indian Railways

10. **The ministry responsible for rehabilitation of the handicapped is called:**
    A. Ministry of Education
    B. Ministry of Labor
    C. Ministry of Home affairs
    D. Ministry of Social Justice and Empowerment

11. **The organization responsible for enforcing uniform standards in training of rehabilitation professionals is:**
    A. National Rehabilitation University
    B. National Association of Rehabilitation Professionals
    C. Rehabilitation Council of India
    D. Apex Rehabilitation Co-ordination Committee

| 6. C | 7. C | 8. C | 9. D | 10. D | 11. C |

Chapter 3: Sociolegal Aspects of Rehabilitation

12. Concessions for the disabled are given in all categories, *except*:
    A. Travel
    B. Food
    C. Postage
    D. Customs exemption for electronic larynx
13. A disability certificate can be issued by the following, *except*:
    A. ENT surgeon
    B. Ophthalmologist
    C. Medical social worker
    D. Physiatrist
14. The travel concession by rail for a blind person is 75% for all categories of travel, *except*:
    A. First class
    B. AC three tier
    C. AC two tier
    D. AC chair car
15. The Rehabilitation Council of India enforces uniform standards in training of professionals in the field of rehabilitation by all of the following, *except*:
    A. Maintains a central rehabilitation register
    B. Regulates standards in educational institutions throughout the country
    C. Does not recognize foreign qualifications
    D. Inspects examinations conducted by training institutions in rehabilitation
16. The formula used for calculating percentage of impairment in multiple disability is (a = higher value, b = lower value)
    A. $a + b(90-b)/90$
    B. $a + b(90-a)/90$
    C. $a + b(b-90)/90$
    D. $a + b(a-90)/90$
17. The percentage of disability in stroke is calculated using:
    A. Modified Barthel scale
    B. Disability rating scale
    C. Modified Rankin scale
    D. McGill stroke scale

12. B	13. C	14. C	15. C	16. B	17. C

18. The rights of the persons with disability (PWD) was passed in:
   A. 2017
   B. 2018
   C. 2016
   D. 2014
19. The maximum % of permanent impairment in relation to that specific limb would be given to a person with:
   A. Amputation through proximal phalanx or disarticulation through MP joint of index finger, middle finger, ring finger and little finger
   B. Amputation through proximal phalanx or disarticulation through MP joint of index finger, middle finger and ring finger
   C. Loss of all toes
   D. Thumb disarticulation through CM joint

18. C 19. D

CHAPTER 4

Architectural Barriers

1. **Telephone adaptation device for profoundly hearing disabled should be provided with a modification such as:**
   A. Adjustable amplifiers
   B. Push button dial
   C. Rotating dial
   D. Flickering lights, when a call comes
2. **Accessibility for disabled children should be made easy by modification of household furnishings as follows:**
   A. Placement of padding at the pointed edges of furniture
   B. Use of safety glass in furniture
   C. Keeping dangerous objects out of reach
   D. All of the above
3. **Old age home for disabled senior citizens should be provided with the following facilities, *except*:**
   A. Simple environmental setting with familiar surroundings
   B. Easy access to toilet or bedroom
   C. Dim lighting so as to not irritate eyes
   D. Provision of spaces for interaction with other residents
4. **The following appliances may be used in case of emergency for severely visually impaired, *except*:**
   A. Exit signs near stair way
   B. Tactile maps
   C. Emergency siren
   D. Vibrating pagers

1. D   2. D   3. C   4. A

5. Modifications to be taken for a locomotor disabled person for the toilet/bathroom are all the following, *except*:
   A. Grab rail along the bath area
   B. Nonslip rubber mat for safety
   C. Indian type of closet is preferred
   D. Bath oils and shampoos that make the floor slippery should be avoided
6. For a severe locomotor disabled patient the toilet/bathroom should have all of the following, *except*:
   A. Anti skid flooring
   B. Good lighting
   C. Hand rails
   D. Bath tub with nonslippery surface
7. In a patient with osteoarthritis hip and knee, the modification of the toilet should be:
   A. Indian style toilet
   B. A western commode
   C. Bed-pan
   D. None of the above
8. The work centers in a kitchen are arranged as follows:
   A. Storage, sink, stove
   B. Sink, storage, stove
   C. Storage, stove, sink
   D. Stove, sink, storage
9. The minimum gradient of slope for a ramp for independent use should be:
   A. 1:2
   B. 1:4
   C. 1:12
   D. 1:6
10. Wet dynamic coefficient of friction on the floor of public spaces used by people with disability should be more than:
    A. 0.012–0.014
    B. 0.12–0.14
    C. 0.042–0.06
    D. 0.4–0.6

| 5. C | 6. D | 7. B | 8. C | 9. C | 10. D |

Chapter 4: Architectural Barriers

11. All of the following statements for disability are true, *except*:
    A. All new public buildings have to be modeled to be barrier free to all disabilities
    B. There must be at least three landings between two floors
    C. Horizontal sliding doors are the easiest to operate from the sitting position
    D. In all new public buildings ramps are constructed in addition to staircases
12. One of the following is hazardous for wheelchair bound individuals:
    A. Glass panels on doors
    B. Horizontal sliding doors
    C. Folding doors
    D. Two way swinging doors
13. One of the following is not a modification for a wheelchair user:
    A. Modifying the height of switches
    B. Ramps
    C. Nontransparent hinged doors
    D. Widening the door
14. One of the following is a specific furniture modification for spastic cerebral diplegia with hip adductor tightness:
    A. Foot rest
    B. Back rest
    C. Pommel
    D. Arm rest
15. One of the following statements is true:
    A. The person with disability (PWD) is seated close to the screen in a movie theater so that he can enjoy the details of the scenes
    B. There should not be any prioritization in allotment of parking lots to PWD
    C. The PWD is seated close to the entrance
    D. Flashing lights are used to alert all people with handicap in cases of emergency
16. The following is a modification for hearing disability:
    A. Hand faucet
    B. Pommel
    C. Vibrating alerts
    D. Braille inscription

11. B 12. D 13. C 14. C 15. C 16. C

Section I: General Principles

17. The following is a modification for visual disability:
    A. Hand faucet
    B. Pommel
    C. Vibrating alerts
    D. Braille inscription
18. The following is a modification for a paraplegic:
    A. Hand faucet
    B. Pommel
    C. Vibrating pager
    D. Braille inscription
19. Self-help aid for a quadriplegic:
    A. Reciprocal walker
    B. Hand rail
    C. Page turner
    D. Wheelchair
20. Environmental modifications to help patients with limited attention capabilities include:
    A. Increasing contrast and maximizing lighting
    B. Keeping everything in its place
    C. Reducing the number of distractors
    D. All of the above
21. Which of the following is not true with regard to home assessment or evaluation?
    A. It is a review of the details of a home environment with attention to barriers to access
    B. Best performed after a new wheelchair user returns home.
    C. Typically includes provision of a floor plan—annotated measurements of all thresholds, room sizes, doorway widths, furniture, appliance and plumbing placements, and elevations such as stairs and ramps
    D. Assess the home for safety and accessibility
22. Examples of environmental modifications include all the following, *except*:
    A. Installation of ramps into buildings
    B. Installation of grab bars for bathroom safety
    C. Arrangement of furniture in the home or at work
    D. Usage of crutches to climb stairs

17. D   18. A   19. C   20. D   21. B   22. D

CHAPTER 5

Activities of Daily Living

1. **Technological innovations to improve accessibility include the following, *except*:**
   A. Environment control systems
   B. Voice controlled wheelchair
   C. Tactile maps to show the direction
   D. Electronic larynx
2. **Modifications to improve accessibility for wheelchair users include the following, *except*:**
   A. Bathroom fixtures design which include hand held showers
   B. Electronically controlled windows
   C. Standing frame
   D. Low set electrical switches
3. **Activities of daily living are needed for:**
   A. Self-maintenance   B. Mobility
   C. Communication   D. All of the above
4. **Instrumental activities of daily living include all, *except*:**
   A. Child rearing
   B. Community mobility
   C. Sexual activity
   D. Meal preparation and cleanup
5. **Which of the following is false?**
   A. Inserting a key uses the lateral pinch
   B. Writing with a pen uses the three jaw chuck pinch
   C. Picking up a pin uses the tip to tip pinch
   D. None of the above

1. D   2. C   3. D   4. C   5. D

Section I: General Principles

6. Environmental control system consists of the following, *except*:
   A. An input method
   B. A control device to change the input into a signal
   C. A receiving device to receive the input signals
   D. EMG biofeedback mechanisms
7. The purpose of an environmental control system is to:
   A. Maximize functional ability and independence
   B. Environment control for climatic change affecting the disabled
   C. Help the person ambulate in the immediate environment
   D. All of the above
8. Training the patient in performing ADL should be based on the following criteria, *except*:
   A. It may be graded by beginning with a few simple tasks and gradually increasing their number and complexity
   B. It must be tailored to suit each patient's learning style and ability
   C. Architectural barriers must be removed at home and office
   D. Fixed protocols should be used for all types of patients
9. Type of clothing recommended for person with upper extremity amputation include the following, *except*:
   A. The clothing should be loose fitting and front fastening
   B. Velcro fasteners for the trousers
   C. Shoes without laces
   D. Buttons instead of zippers for shirts
10. Environmental adaptations for better hygiene and grooming include the following, *except*:
    A. A brush with grip is used for bathing or shampooing hair
    B. A long handled bath brush
    C. Dressing sticks to enable the person to pull on clothes
    D. Head pointer
11. Home management tips for a person with severe rheumatoid arthritis include the following, *except*:
    A. Use a reacher to get items
    B. Store frequently used items on higher shelves of the cabinet for safety
    C. Use light weight utensils
    D. Use long handled taps

6. D   7. A   8. D   9. D   10. D   11. B

Chapter 5: Activities of Daily Living

12. **Communication adaptations include following, *except*:**
    A. Eye tracking systems
    B. Built up pens and pencils with an easier grip
    C. Speech to text software
    D. Voice activated motorized wheelchair
13. **Pushing a table is an example of:**
    A. Prehensile movement
    B. Nonprehensile movement
    C. Protective movement
    D. Manipulative movement
14. **Release of an object in a hook grip is accomplished by:**
    A. Relaxation of either extensors or the flexors of the hand
    B. Relaxation of the flexors followed by contraction of the finger extensors
    C. Contraction of both flexors and extensors of the fingers
    D. None of the above
15. **In activities involving both upper limbs very often the stabilizing function of the hand is carried out by:**
    A. Dominant hand
    B. Nondominant hand
    C. Both of the above
    D. Shoulder
16. **Following are included in gross motor abilities, *except*:**
    A. Holding a cup
    B. Threading a needle
    C. Changing tyres of a car
    D. Holding a book
17. **Precautions taken for the patient with sensory impairment include all the following, *except*:**
    A. Safer handling of sharp objects
    B. Regular observation for skin changes
    C. Care during handling of hot objects
    D. Keeping the extremities moist

12. D   13. B   14. B   15. B   16. B   17. D

Section I: General Principles

18. Activities of daily living include all, *except*:
    A. Bathing and showering
    B. Communication device use
    C. Dressing
    D. Feeding
19. Any equipment or product system whether acquired commercially off the shelf, modified, or customized that is used to increase or improve functional capabilities of individuals with disabilities is known as:
    A. Assistive device
    B. Orthotics
    C. ADL
    D. Mobility aids
20. _____ is used as an outcome measure for activities of daily living:
    A. Functional activity index (FAI)
    B. Barthel index
    C. Occupational therapy measure
    D. Tardieu scale

18. B   19. A   20. B

II Therapeutic Management

SECTION OUTLINE

6. Therapeutic Exercises and Techniques
7. Clinical Examination
8. Gait
9. Hand Function and Occupational Therapy
10. Management of Communication Impairment
11. Management of Behavioral and Learning Problems
12. Orthotics
13. Prosthetics
14. Mobility Aids
15. Vocational Rehabilitation
16. Pain and Musculoskeletal Disorders
17. Surgery in Rehabilitation
18. Physical Agents

CHAPTER 6

Therapeutic Exercises and Techniques

1. **Benefits of continuous passive movement include all, *except*:**
   A. Increase range of movement in postoperative cases of knee replacement or ACL reconstruction
   B. Reduces pain in flexion of the knee in septic arthritis
   C. Prevents development of contractures
   D. Increases blood supply to the joint
2. **What do you mean by proprioceptive neuromuscular facilitation?**
   A. The application of deep stretches to the musculotendinous unit resulting in increased flexibility of muscles and range of motion
   B. Actual production of movement response and implies reaching a critical threshold level for neuronal activity
   C. Decreased capacity to initiate a movement response through the altered synaptic potential
   D. Facilitation of an electrical signal in the muscle to change its resting potential
3. **The steady contraction of muscles that is necessary to hold different parts of the skeleton in proper relation to each other in various attitudes of the body:**
   A. Opisthotonus   B. Hypertension
   C. Postural tone   D. Flexor synergy
4. **Exercises performed by the patient by himself or herself are all the following, *except*:**
   A. Active exercises   B. Passive exercises
   C. Resisted exercises D. Coordination exercises

1. B   2. A   3. C   4. B

Section II: Therapeutic Management

5. The application of a maintained external force to stretch a body segment is referred to as:
   A. Facilitated stretching
   B. Passive stretching
   C. Selective stretching
   D. None of the above
6. Which of the following is characteristic of closed kinetic chain exercises?
   A. More shear stress created
   B. Distal end fixed
   C. Leg extension with free weights
   D. Frenkels exercises
7. All the following are done for a recovering stroke patient, *except*:
   A. Position the patient to avoid pressure sore, contracture and overstretching of joint structures
   B. Change the position once in two hours from affected side to unaffected side and to supine
   C. Have a height adjustable bed to enable easy transfer
   D. Position the bed in such a way that the patient can use his normal side for all his needs
8. Following are the methods to reduce spasticity, *except*:
   A. Application of long icing
   B. Apply reflex inhibiting postures
   C. Slow stretch to the spastic muscles
   D. Giving noxious stimuli to stimulate sensory cortex
9. The rehabilitation technique used to stimulate the neuromuscular system in an effort to excite proprioceptors:
   A. Neuromuscular electric stimulation
   B. Rood's technique
   C. Alexander technique
   D. PNF techniques
10. Another term for percussion is:
    A. Effleurage
    B. Petrissage
    C. Tapotement
    D. Stroking

5. B   6. B   7. D   8. D   9. D   10. C

Chapter 6: Therapeutic Exercises and Techniques

11. **What type of exercise should be avoided in patients with osteoporotic compression fractures?**
    A. Walking
    B. Spinal flexion exercises
    C. Progressive resistive back extension exercises
    D. Swimming
12. **In knee extension lag, the person will be able to do all, *except*:**
    A. Do knee bending activities
    B. Perform straight leg raising test
    C. Sit cross legged
    D. All of the above
13. **The flexion synergy in the lower limb includes:**
    A. Hip flexion, abduction and external rotation
    B. Hip flexion, adduction and external rotation
    C. Hip flexion, abduction and internal rotation
    D. Hip flexion, adduction and internal rotation
14. **In osteoarthritis of the knee, the area most commonly affected is:**
    A. Posterior compartment
    B. Lateral compartment
    C. Medial compartment
    D. Anterolateral compartment
15. **Which of the following statements is NOT true regarding facet joint-mediated pain?**
    A. Rehabilitation should be focused on exercises with neutral or flexion posture to reduce stress on facet joints
    B. Diagnostic use of facet joint nerve blocks and therapeutic radiofrequency ablation are treatment options
    C. To minimize the false-positive response that occurs with one injection, two separate blocks using different-duration anesthetics are recommended
    D. Facet joint-mediated pain is likely to be elicited on flexion or repetitive end-range flexion
16. **Which of the following is characteristic of open kinetic chain exercises?**
    A. Distal end fixed   B. Squatting
    C. Less shear stress   D. Distal end not fixed

11. B   12. B   13. A   14. C   15. D   16. D

Section II: Therapeutic Management

17. Which of the following exercises is recommended for rheumatoid arthritis?
    A. Isotonic
    B. Concentric
    C. Isokinetic
    D. Isometric
18. If the patient is able to move his knee in full range parallel to ground then what is the power of his quadriceps?
    A. 1
    B. Equal to or less than 2
    C. 3
    D. Equal to or more than 2
19. Maximum power is generated in which range of muscle contraction?
    A. Inner range
    B. Middle range
    C. Outer range
    D. None of the above
20. The term kinesiology refers to:
    A. The force vector producing forward movement of the center of gravity of the body
    B. The study of the principles of mechanics and anatomy in relation to human movement
    C. Movement between articular surfaces of the joints
    D. Analysis of the speed of movement of the body
21. What do you mean by plasticity of soft tissue?
    A. The point on the soft tissue where fatigue occurs after a stretching force
    B. The quality of soft tissue that allows it to maintain a lengthened state after a stretch force has been removed
    C. The point where the tissue will return to its original position when stretch force is removed
    D. The breaking point of the soft tissue when the stretch force is applied continuously

17. D   18. D   19. B   20. B   21. B

Chapter 6: Therapeutic Exercises and Techniques

22. **Which of the following exercises would be contraindicated in a patient with ankylosing spondylitis?**
    A. Range of motion exercises
    B. Stretching and strengthening
    C. Spinal extensors strengthening exercises
    D. Spinal flexion exercises
23. **Close packed position of glenohumeral joint:**
    A. Abduction and internal rotation
    B. Abduction and external rotation
    C. Flexion and internal rotation
    D. Adduction and lateral rotation
24. **When the muscle shortens, the muscle is said to be working_____.**
    A. Concentrically
    B. Eccentrically
    C. Isometrically
    D. None of the above
25. **Goal of giving PROM is:**
    A. Maintain joint mobility
    B. Prevention of contractures
    C. Maintain connective tissue mobility
    D. All of the above
26. **Physiological effects of active range of motion exercises are all, *except*:**
    A. To maintain elasticity of participating muscles
    B. To provide sensory feedback from the contracting muscles
    C. To enhance contraction of smooth muscle fibers
    D. To improve coordination and motor skills

22. D   23. B   24. A   25. D   26. C

CHAPTER 7

Clinical Examination

1. **Lachman test of knee is done to indicate integrity of:**
   A. Medial ligament
   B. Lateral ligament
   C. Anterior cruciate ligament
   D. All of the above
2. **Barlow's sign is diagnostic of:**
   A. Tuberculosis of hip
   B. Legg-Perthes disease
   C. DDH
   D. Osteoarthritis hip
3. **Trendelenburg test is done to test which group of hip muscles:**
   A. Flexors
   B. Extensors
   C. Adductors
   D. Abductors
4. **Which test is carried out for testing the hip flexor tightness?**
   A. Thomas test
   B. Ober's test
   C. Faber's test
   D. Ely's test
5. **Flexor tightness of the knee is tested with hip:**
   A. Extended and knee flexed
   B. Flexed and knee extended
   C. Abducted and knee flexed
   D. Adducted and knee extended

1. C   2. C   3. D   4. A   5. B

6. The Sweep test is performed for:
   A. Spinal flexion
   B. Knee joint effusion
   C. Perthes disease
   D. Osteoarthritis of wrist
7. Winging of scapula is usually due to paralysis of which muscle?
   A. Serratus anterior
   B. Levator scapulae
   C. Latissimus dorsi
   D. Supraspinatus
8. If you give a noxious stimulus at the sole of the foot what kind of response will be seen in a child?
   A. Cross extension
   B. Flexor withdrawal
   C. Extensor thrust
   D. Landau reflex
9. One of the tests of integrity of radial nerve is:
   A. Ulnar deviation
   B. Flexion of semiprone elbow
   C. Wrist and finger flexion
   D. Card test
10. Loss of opposition of the thumb is due to injury of:
    A. Radial nerve
    B. Ulnar nerve
    C. Median nerve
    D. Axillary nerve
11. Common neurological signs in Bell's palsy include the following, *except*:
    A. Inability to close the ipsilateral eye
    B. Loss of taste on the anterior 2/3rds of the tongue
    C. Eye will be closed with lateral deviation of eyeball
    D. Diminished nasolabial fold
12. A patient lifts his hip and bends his knee in an exaggerated fashion to clear the ground. This is called:
    A. Circumduction gait   B. Quadriceps gait
    C. Festinant gait   D. High steppage gait

6. B   7. A   8. B   9. B   10. C   11. C   12. D

Section II: Therapeutic Management

13. **Cogwheel and lead pipe are types of:**
    A. Abnormal movements
    B. Rigidity
    C. Tremor
    D. Flaccidity
14. **Bradykinesia is:**
    A. Cramped writing
    B. Tremor
    C. Slowness of movement
    D. Expressionless face
15. **Difficulty to perform rapid alternating movements is known as:**
    A. Dysmetria
    B. Dysdiadochokinesia
    C. Bradykinesia
    D. Friedreich's ataxia
16. **Yergasons test is performed to test:**
    A. Triceps
    B. Biceps
    C. Supraspinatus
    D. Infraspinatus
17. **The following statements about nystagmus are true, *except*:**
    A. Most people with nystagmus have some useful vision
    B. Normally nystagmus does not get worse with age
    C. It never presents in childhood
    D. None of the above
18. **Hemiballismus results from a lesion of contralateral:**
    A. Subthalamic nucleus
    B. Cortical center No. 34
    C. Putamen
    D. Red nucleus
19. **Opisthotonus is sustained contraction of:**
    A. Flexor muscles of neck and trunk
    B. Extensor muscles of neck and trunk
    C. Trunk rotators
    D. Sternocleidomastoid

13. B   14. C   15. B   16. B   17. C   18. A   19. B

Chapter 7: Clinical Examination

20. **Fasciculations are spontaneous potentials seen with:**
    A. Irritation of anterior horn cell
    B. Degeneration of nerve roots
    C. Muscle spasm or cramps
    D. All of the above
21. **Painful arc syndrome or sign is to diagnose:**
    A. Bicipital tendinitis
    B. Shoulder impingement
    C. Lateral rotation of neck
    D. Adhesive capsulitis
22. **Cozen's test is done for:**
    A. Supraspinatus tendinitis
    B. Triceps tendinitis
    C. Lateral epicondylitis
    D. Subacromial bursitis
23. **Finkelstein's test is done for:**
    A. Supraspinatus
    B. De Quervain's tenosynovitis
    C. Golfers elbow
    D. None of the above
24. **Adson maneuver is to test vascular compromise of:**
    A. Femoral artery
    B. Brachial artery
    C. Subclavian artery
    D. Common carotid artery
25. **Abduction of the 5th digit, with the inability to adduct it is:**
    A. Ortolanis sign
    B. De Quervain's sign
    C. Wartenberg's sign
    D. Finkelstein's sign

20. D   21. B   22. C   23. B   24. C   25. C

CHAPTER

8

Gait

1. Which of the following is non-weight bearing gait (on any one of the lower limbs)?
   A. Three point gait pattern
   B. Two point gait pattern
   C. Four point gait pattern
   D. None of the above
2. The distance between the right heel strike followed by left heel strike in a gait cycle is known as:
   A. Right step length
   B. Left step length
   C. Right stride length
   D. Left stride length
3. Hand-knee gait is commonly due to:
   A. Weakness of hamstrings muscle
   B. Weakness of quadriceps muscle
   C. Weakness of plantar flexors
   D. Lack of balance on that side
4. Ataxic gait is often due to a lesion in the:
   A. Motor area   B. Basal ganglia
   C. Pons   D. Cerebellum
5. Two crutches in contact with the floor in front of the body and moving both limbs past the crutches describes which crutch gait?
   A. Two-point gait   B. Three-point gait
   C. Swing-through gait D. Swing-to gait

1. A   2. B   3. B   4. D   5. C

6. Two crutches in contact with the floor in front of the body and moving both limbs almost to the level of the crutches describes which crutch gait?
   A. Two-point gait
   B. Three-point gait
   C. Swing-through gait
   D. Swing-to gait
7. One crutch and opposite extremity moving together followed by the other crutch and other extremity describes which crutch gait?
   A. Two-point gait
   B. Three-point gait
   C. Swing-through gait
   D. Swing-to gait
8. The linear distance between corresponding successive points of contact of the same foot (e.g., distance measured from heel strike to heel strike of the same foot) in the gait cycle is known as:
   A. Step length
   B. Stride length
   C. Cadence
   D. Stance
9. The time period in the gait cycle during which the limb is in contact with the ground is called:
   A. Swing phase
   B. Stance phase
   C. Initial contact
   D. Loading response
10. Components of stance phase are all of the following, *except*:
    A. Initial contact
    B. Terminal swing
    C. Preswing [toe off]
    D. Loading response
11. The determinants of gait are all of the following, *except*:
    A. Pelvic rotation
    B. Pelvic tilt
    C. Foot and knee mechanisms
    D. Knee extension in stance phase

6. D   7. A   8. B   9. B   10. B   11. D

Section II: Therapeutic Management

12. The center of gravity (COG) of the body is typically located:
    A. 5 cm in front of the lumbosacral junction
    B. 5 cm posterior to the body of the S2 vertebra
    C. 5 cm anterior to the S2 vertebra
    D. In front of the first sacral vertebra
13. Foot drop or foot slap and a high steppage gait maybe due to weakness of all of the following, *except*:
    A. Tibialis anterior
    B. EDL
    C. EHL
    D. Tendo-Achilles
14. Muscles that need strengthening in preparation for crutch walking are all, *except*:
    A. Latissimus dorsi
    B. Triceps
    C. Pectoralis major
    D. Trapezius
15. The normal distribution of time during the gait cycle at normal walking speed is:
    A. 60% for stance phase and 40% for swing phase
    B. 40% for stance phase and 60% for swing phase
    C. 80% for stance phase and 20% for swing phase
    D. 20% for stance phase and 80% for swing phase
16. The gait of a person with bilateral adductor tightness is:
    A. Trendelenburg gait
    B. Scissoring gait
    C. Swaying gait
    D. Crouch gait
17. The Trendelenburg gait is due to weakness of:
    A. Gluteus maximus
    B. Long flexors of the hip
    C. Extensors of the hip
    D. Gluteus medius

12. C   13. D   14. D   15. A   16. B   17. D

18. When a patient walks with pain in one or both lower extremities it is called:
    A. Waddling gait
    B. Stamping gait
    C. Antalgic gait
    D. Algic gait
19. Foot drop or foot slap and a high steppage gait maybe due to paralysis of:
    A. Sural nerve
    B. Lateral cutaneous nerve
    C. Femoral nerve
    D. Peroneal nerve

18. C   19. D

CHAPTER 9

Hand Function and Occupational Therapy

1. **Hand grasp strength is measured with:**
   A. Pinch gauge
   B. Dynamometer
   C. Muscle testing
   D. Sensory evoked potentials
2. **To check fine motor hand function you need to check the:**
   A. Grasp
   B. Pinch
   C. Proprioception
   D. Protection
3. **Ambidexterity is:**
   A. Usage of right hand as dominant
   B. Usage of left hand as dominant
   C. Usage of both hands equally
   D. None of the above
4. **Precision work does not involve:**
   A. Tip to tip pinch
   B. Palmar pinch
   C. Lateral pinch
   D. Hookgrip
5. **The following are grips, *except*:**
   A. Cylindrical
   B. Pulp
   C. Spherical
   D. Hook

1. B   2. B   3. C   4. D   5. B

Chapter 9: Hand Function and Occupational Therapy

6. **Functional position of the hand is:**
   A. Wrist extension, MCP extension, IP flexion, thumb adduction
   B. Wrist extension, MCP extension, IP flexion, thumb abduction
   C. Wrist extension, MCP flexion, IP extension, thumb in opposition
   D. Wrist extension, MCP flexion, IP flexion, thumb abduction
7. **A distorted representation of different parts of the human body based on a "map" of the areas in the brain, dedicated to processing motor or sensory functions, is called:**
   A. Gyri and sulci of the cortex
   B. Neurological mapping
   C. Cortical homunculus
   D. Motor and sensory centers
8. **FOOSH stands for:**
   A. Functional operation for occupational safety and health
   B. Facilitation in occupational overuse syndrome in hands
   C. Fall on outstretched hand
   D. Function of occupational splinting of hand
9. **If a persons entire radius, ulna, carpals, metacarpals, and phalanges are removed, he has had:**
   A. Below the elbow   B. Above the elbow
   C. Mid elbow   D. Elbow disarticulation
10. **Humans can perform the following grip which a monkey cannot:**
    A. Hook grip
    B. Three jaw-chuck pinch
    C. Cylindrical grip
    D. None of the above
11. **If you were to carry a heavy suitcase, you would use:**
    A. Power grasp   B. Heavy duty grasp
    C. Hook pattern   D. Spherical grasp
12. **Which of the following body actions (among others) will activate the terminal device on an upper extremity prosthesis?**
    A. Scapular abduction   B. Shoulder extension
    C. Chest contraction   D. Elbow extension

6. D   7. C   8. C   9. D   10. B   11. C   12. A

Section II: Therapeutic Management

13. **The swan neck splint allows for:**
    A. Flexion at the PIP joint and flexion of the DIP joint
    B. Flexion at the PIP joint and prevents extension at DIP joints
    C. Extension of the PIP joint and flexion of the DIP joint
    D. Flexion and extension at the PIP joint, but only extension at the DIP joint

14. **The ideal shape of the upper extremity residual limb (AE) is:**
    A. Cylindrical
    B. Conical
    C. Tapered
    D. None of the above

15. **The goal for hand positioning to prevent the development of a "claw" hand deformity, is:**
    A. Wrist joint flexed, MCP joint flexed, PIP joint flexed, DIP joint extended
    B. Wrist joint extended, MCP joint extended, PIP joint and, DIP joint flexed
    C. Wrist joint flexed, MCP joint extended, PIP joint extended, DIP extended
    D. Wrist extended, MCP joint flexed, PIP joint extended, DIP joint extended

16. **The term prehensile refers to:**
    A. Training to do fine motor movements
    B. Grasp by wrapping around of the fingers
    C. Poor cylindrical grip
    D. Fear or apprehension of gripping

17. **The nerve passing through the carpal tunnel into the hand is:**
    A. Nerve to abductor digiti minimi
    B. The median nerve
    C. The ulnar nerve
    D. The radial nerve

18. **A rupture of the terminal extensor tendon of the distal phalanx of the finger can cause:**
    A. Swan neck deformity
    B. Z shaped deformity
    C. Mallet finger
    D. None of the above

13. B 14. A 15. D 16. B 17. B 18. C

Chapter 9: Hand Function and Occupational Therapy

19. De Quervain's tenosynovitis affects the:
    A. Extensor pollicis brevis (EPB) and flexor digitorum superficialis (FDS)
    B. Adductor pollicis brevis (APB) and extensor digitorum profundus (FDP)
    C. Flexor digitorum superficialis (FCR) and abductor pollicis longus (APL)
    D. Extensor pollicis brevis (EPB) and abductor pollicis longus (APL)
20. Boxer's fractures involve a fracture of which bone?
    A. Scaphoid
    B. Hamate
    C. First metacarpal
    D. Fifth metacarpal
21. The nerves most commonly affecting a pincer grasp, as in operating a knob on a stove is:
    A. Ulnar nerve
    B. Radial nerve
    C. Median nerve
    D. All of the above
22. A weighted spoon for feeding would be most useful for a person suffering from:
    A. Parkinson's disease
    B. Quadriplegia
    C. Osteoarthritis of the fingers
    D. All of the above
23. Which of the following orthoses closes the hand of a tetraplegic using wrist extension?
    A. Knuckle bender orthosis
    B. Wrist orthosis
    C. Tenodesis orthosis
    D. Long opponens orthosis
24. The thumb is not used in:
    A. Span grip
    B. Key pinch
    C. Hook grip
    D. Cylindrical grip

19. D   20. D   21. C   22. A   23. C   24. C

CHAPTER

10

Management of Communication Impairment

1. **Perceptually distinct units of sound in a specified language that distinguish one word from another, are:**
   A. Consonants   B. Words
   C. Vowels   D. Phonemes
2. **In English, the pronunciation of the letters *p b* and *m* is.**
   A. Labiodental B. Bilabial
   C. Alveolar   D. Palatal
3. **The speech receptive area of the brain is called:**
   A. Broca's area
   B. Wernicke's area
   C. Temporoparietal lobe
   D. Arcuate fasciculus
4. **Transcortical motor aphasia is different from Broca's aphasia in that:**
   A. Ability to speak fluently in jargon language is present in transcortical aphasia
   B. Ability to understand only single stage commands in transcortical aphasia
   C. Ability to repeat frequently is present in transcortical aphasia
   D. Ability to identify items by name is present
5. **A person who speaks quite fluently with good comprehension but cannot repeat suffers from:**
   A. Transcortical sensory aphasia
   B. Anomic aphasia
   C. Isolation aphasia
   D. Conduction aphasia

| 1. D | 2. B | 3. B | 4. C | 5. D |

Chapter 10: Management of Communication Impairment

6. **The following person qualifies for test of communication impairment:**
   A. Mentally retarded person
   B. Profoundly schizophrenic
   C. Completely illiterate
   D. Dysarthria
7. **Combination of flaccid and spastic dysarthria may occur in:**
   A. Amyotrophic lateral sclerosis
   B. Bulbar polio
   C. Stroke
   D. Cerebellar lesions
8. **Scanning speech is seen in:**
   A. Flaccid dysarthria
   B. Cerebellar dysarthria
   C. Bulbar poliomyelitis
   D. Spastic dysarthria
9. **Lack of sound/voice during speech is:**
   A. Aphasia   B. Laryngomalacia
   C. Aphonia   D. Pubophonia
10. **An augmentative communication device consists of all, *except*:**
    A. Interface
    B. Input device
    C. Wireless aided communication system (WACS)
    D. Output device
11. **Stimuli are transmitted to the external ear through head phones to test:**
    A. Bone conduction
    B. Air conduction
    C. None of the above
    D. Both A and B above
12. **The Snellen's chart measures:**
    A. Visual acuity
    B. Colour vision
    C. Intraocular pressure
    D. Hypermetropia

6. D   7. A   8. B   9. C   10. C   11. B   12. A

Section II: Therapeutic Management

13. A Braille cell consists of dots in:
    A. Two columns and two rows
    B. Two columns and three rows
    C. Three columns and three rows
    D. Three columns and two rows
14. The definition of deafness (hearing impairment) as stipulated in the RPWD Act, 2016 is a person who has a minimum of _____ of hearing impairment in both ears in speech conversation frequencies:
    A. 70 B. 55
    C. 60 D. 50
15. Dysphagia is defined as:
    A. Communication disorder characterized by impairment of language comprehension, formulation and use
    B. Motor speech defects lead to slurring, slow speech, prolonged pauses or uneven stress on syllables
    C. Lack of appetite
    D. Any defect in the intake or transport of endogenous secretions and necessary food for maintenance of life
16. Dysarthria is defined as:
    A. Communication disorder characterized by impairment of language comprehension, formulation and use
    B. Motor speech defects that lead to slurring, slow speech, prolonged pauses or uneven stress on syllables
    C. Disturbed language development as well as disrupted use of interactive skills
    D. Lack of voice production
17. Broca's aphasia occurs due to lesion at:
    A. Area No. 44   B. Area No. 23
    C. Area No. 27   D. None of the above
18. Blindness is defined by the RPWD Act 2016 as under the following, *except*:
    A. Color blindness for at least one color in the visual spectrum
    B. Inability of a person to count fingers from a distance of 6 meters or 20 feet (technical definition)
    C. Vision 6/60 or less with the best possible spectacle correction
    D. Diminution of field vision to 20 feet or less in better eye

13. B   14. C   15. D   16. B   17. A   18. A

Chapter 10: Management of Communication Impairment

19. The normal human ear perceives simple tones in the range of:
    A. 20-20,000 Hz
    B. 200-20000 Hz
    C. 20-2000 Hz
    D. 200-2000 Hz
20. Presenting stimuli with vibrator on mastoid process is done to test:
    A. Bone conduction
    B. Air conduction
    C. None of the above
    D. Both A and B
21. Defective articulation but with the content of speech unaffected refers to:
    A. Verbal apraxia
    B. Nominal aphasia
    C. Dysarthria
    D. Aphasia
22. In the general population, aphasia usually results due to cortical lesions of the:
    A. Hypothalamus
    B. Occipital lobe
    C. Left hemisphere
    D. Cerebellum
23. Aphasia is an impairment of:
    A. Comprehension
    B. Memory
    C. Phonation
    D. Language
24. The language disorder that results from damage to the arcuate fasciculus is called:
    A. Broca's aphasia   B. Wernicke's aphasia
    C. Conduction aphasia D. Global aphasia
25. Wernicke's area is in Brodmanns area number:
    A. 25   B. 44
    C. 22   D. 41

19. A   20. A   21. C   22. C   23. D   24. C   25. C

CHAPTER

11

Management of Behavioral and Learning Problems

1. **The fright and flight response is an example of:**
   A. Operant behavior
   B. Security response
   C. Respondent behavior
   D. Emotional response
2. **Mental illness associated with impaired brain tissue function is:**
   A. Functional psychosis B. Organic psychosis
   C. Tactile hallucination D. Hysteria
3. **Unexplained fears of situation, objects is called as:**
   A. Delusion   B. Illusion
   C. Neurosis   D. Phobia
4. **Which of the following can occur in normal persons?**
   A. Illusion   B. Delusion
   C. Conversion reaction D. Neurosis
5. **Which of the following is true?**
   A. The frequency of behavior occurrence is inversely proportional to a positive reinforcer
   B. The frequency of behavior occurrence is inversely proportional to a negative reinforcer
   C. The frequency of behavior occurrence is directly proportional to a negative reinforcer
   D. The frequency of behavior occurrence is not proportional to a negative reinforce but only to positive reinforcer

1. C   2. B   3. D   4. A   5. B

Chapter 11: Management of Behavioral and Learning Problems

6. The following are methods used by the special educator, *except*:
   A. Repetition
   B. Inhibition of response
   C. Concretization
   D. Making units of study smaller
7. One of these is not present in autism:
   A. Repetitive activities
   B. Unusual sensory responses
   C. Reduced vision and hearing
   D. Resistance to environmental change
8. The following conditions can predispose to mental retardation, *except*:
   A. Hydrocephaly
   B. Mongolism
   C. Poliomyelitis
   D. Cretinism
9. Dementia is defined as:
   A. Chronic progressive deterioration of intellect, memory and communication
   B. Disorder of articulation
   C. Group of speech disorders resulting from disturbance of motor control
   D. Lack of response due to poor sensory inputs
10. What do you mean by cognition?
    A. Ability of brain to process, store, and manipulate information
    B. Integration of ideas
    C. Constant observation of objects
    D. Registering images on the retina
11. One of the following does not belong to evaluation of cognition:
    A. Attention
    B. Orientation
    C. Memory
    D. Two point discrimination

6. B   7. C   8. C   9. A   10. A   11. D

Section II: Therapeutic Management

12. Aids and strategies for coping with memory impairment include these, *except*:
    A. Personal organizer
    B. Mnemonics
    C. Bliss symbols
    D. Alarms and reminders
13. Lack of memory is known as:
    A. Amnesia
    B. Dyslexia
    C. Dysgraphia
    D. Agnosia
14. Attention deficit hyperactivity disorder (ADHD) is a childhood disorder that is classified under:
    A. Hypokinetic disorders
    B. Hyperactivity disorders
    C. Hyperkinetic disorders
    D. Hyperstasis disorders
15. Which of the following are risk factors for children's psychiatric disorders?
    A. Parental psychopathology
    B. Repeated early separation from parents
    C. Harsh or inadequate parents
    D. All of the above
16. Children with ADHD are known to have deficits in which of the following brain areas?
    A. Perception
    B. Motor functioning
    C. Executive functioning
    D. Memory
17. Children with ADHD are known to have deficits in executive functioning, and specifically have difficulty inhibiting responses. Which of the following brain areas normally controls these types of functions?
    A. The thalamus
    B. The amygdala
    C. The parietal lobes
    D. The frontal lobes

12. C   13. A   14. C   15. D   16. C   17. D

Chapter 11: Management of Behavioral and Learning Problems

18. Teaching parents to identify and reward positive behavior also helps to prevent the child from focusing on the negative and disruptive behaviors generally exhibited by children with both ADHD and conduct disorder. This can be achieved through:
    A. Time out from positive reinforcement
    B. Systemic family therapy
    C. Behavior management techniques
    D. Parent training programs
19. Which of the following teaches parents a range of techniques for controlling and managing their children's symptoms, especially with children diagnosed with conduct disorder?
    A. Systemic family therapy
    B. Functional family therapy
    C. Parent training programs
    D. All of the above
20. Which of the following is a technique that can be used with younger children who are less able to communicate and express their feelings verbally?
    A. Play therapy
    B. Cognitive behavior therapy
    C. Systemic family therapy
    D. Psychodynamic therapy
21. The quality of life of people with intellectual disabilities can be improved significantly with the help of basic training procedures that will equip then with a range of skills depending on their level of disability. The application of learning theory to training in these areas is also known as:
    A. Applied cognitive approaches
    B. Applied treatment analysis
    C. Cognitive behavioral therapy
    D. Applied behavior analysis
22. Dyslexia affects what?
    A. Ability to play sports
    B. Eating
    C. Being able to speak
    D. Reading and learning

18. B   19. C   20. A   21. D   22. D

Section II: Therapeutic Management

23. Which areas are affected by autism?
    A. Cognitive
    B. Behavior
    C. Social interaction
    D. Communication
    E. All of the above
24. Which one would not be considered to be an indicator of learning disorder (LD)?
    A. Problem with math skills
    B. Poor coordination
    C. Difficulty remembering
    D. Limited English proficiency
25. Dyscalculia is a LD associated with:
    A. Fine motor skills
    B. Math skills
    C. Language skills
    D. All of the above
26. Autism is considered as a:
    A. Spectrum with unknown cause
    B. Purely heredity disorder
    C. Lifestyle disability
    D. Due to the environment
27. Which of the following is an example of a specific learning disability (SLD)?
    A. Intellectual disability (mental retardation)
    B. ADHD
    C. Dyslexia
    D. ASD
28. Reading disorder is a developmental disorder and is characterized by reading achievement (e.g., accuracy, speed and comprehension) being significantly below standards expected for which of the following:
    A. Chronological age
    B. IQ
    C. School experience
    D. All of the above

23. E   24. D   25. B   26. A   27. C   28. D

Chapter 11: Management of Behavioral and Learning Problems

29. Which of the following might occur in expressive language disorder?
    a. Limited amount of speech
    b. Difficulty finding the right word
    c. Difficulty new words
    d. All of the above
30. Which of the following is not a physical cause normally associated with phonological disorder?
    a. Hearing impairment
    b. Cleft palate
    c. Small frontal lobes
    d. Cerebral palsy
31. Which of the following is a technique used to address stuttering?
    a. Purposeful speech
    b. Practical speech
    c. Prolonged speech
    d. Delayed speech
32. Fragile X syndrome is associated with which of the following?
    a. Language impairment
    b. Behavioral problems
    c. Moderate levels of intellectual disability
    d. All of the above

29. D   30. C   31. C   32. D

CHAPTER 12

Orthotics

1. **Crutch palsy is due to damage of:**
   A. Median nerve
   B. Radial nerve
   C. Ulnar nerve
   D. Long thoracic nerve
2. **The function of an orthosis is all the following, *except*:**
   A. Support
   B. Stabilization
   C. Immobilization
   D. Replacement
3. **Internal medial heel wedge is given for:**
   A. Flexible pes planus
   B. Flexible pes varus
   C. Metatarsalgia
   D. Pes equinus
4. **Pavlik harness is given for the correction of:**
   A. Deformities in poliomyelitis
   B. Arthrogryphosis multiplex congenita
   C. DDH developmental dysplasia of the hip
   D. Von Recklinghausen's disease
5. **Floor reaction orthosis is given for weakness of:**
   A. Hamstring muscle
   B. Quadriceps muscle
   C. Hip flexors
   D. Hip extensors

1. B 2. D 3. A 4. C 5. B

6. SOMI brace is given to the patient suffering from:
   A. Scoliosis
   B. Fracture of cervical vertebra
   C. Intervertebral lumbar disc disease
   D. Clavicular fractures
7. The following may be taken into consideration when choosing the ideal material used in an orthosis, *except*:
   A. It should not irritate the skin
   B. It should be cheap
   C. It should be heavy because it has to support the body
   D. It should be easy to maintain
8. What kind of stop is given at the ankle joint in an orthosis for lateral popliteal nerve palsy?
   A. Dorsiflexion stop
   B. Limited motion stop
   C. No motion stop
   D. Plantar flexion stop
9. To prevent pes calcaneus deformity, the following movement should be restricted:
   A. Inversion
   B. Eversion
   C. Plantar flexion
   D. Dorsiflexion
10. In presence of foot drop, what kind of assist is given in the ankle joint of the orthosis?
    A Dorsiflexion assist
    B. Plantar flexion assist
    C. Double action ankle assist
    D. Inversion-eversion assist
11. Medial T strap is given in the orthosis to correct:
    A. Varus
    B. Valgus
    C. Cavus
    D. Equinus
12. In which knee joint does the patients line of gravity fall anterior to the anatomical knee joint, stabilizing the knee during stance phase:
    A. Straight set knee joint
    B. Adjustable knee joint
    C. Posterior offset knee joint
    D. Anterior offset knee joint

6. B   7. C   8. D   9. D   10. A   11. B   12. C

Section II: Therapeutic Management

13. **What type of brace is given for growing children with dynamic scoliosis?**
    A. Milwaukee brace
    B. SOMI brace
    C. Knight brace
    D. None of the above

14. **An example of thoracolumbosacral orthosis is:**
    A. Minnesota brace
    B. SOMI brace
    C. Knight brace
    D. Four poster collar

15. **An example of an orthosis used in radial nerve injury:**
    A. Posterior tube splint
    B. Knuckle bender splint
    C. Frog splint
    D. Dynamic cock up splint

16. **In the three point principle of Jordan the:**
    A. Counter forces are above the central force
    B. Counter forces are distal to the central force
    C. Counter forces are proximal to the central force
    D. Central force is in one direction while the other two counterforces are distal and proximal to it in the opposite direction

17. **All are contraindications to orthoses, *except*:**
    A. Severe intractable deformity
    B. If it limits movements in other normal joints
    C. Diabetes mellitus
    D. Severe skin infection

18. **The following are materials used in the manufacture of orthoses, *except*:**
    A. Aluminium
    B. Plastic
    C. Carbon fiber
    D. Copper alloy

19. **The part of the shoe absent in CTEV boot is:**
    A. Lace stay
    B. Outer border
    C. Heel
    D. Throat

13. A 14. C 15. D 16. D 17. C 18. D 19. C

Chapter 12: Orthotics

20. The part of the shoe to be modified in the case of hallux valgus is:
    A. Toe box
    B. Heel counter
    C. Toe spring
    D. Tongue
21. **High toe box is given in:**
    A. Metatarsalgia
    B. Plantar fascitis
    C. Pes varus
    D. Hammer toes
22. The most common lower limb orthoses among the following, given to a patient with stroke:
    A. KAFO
    B. AFO
    C. HKAFO
    D. All of the above
23. What type of static splint should be given for the patient suffering from tenosynovitis of APL and EPB?
    A. Knuckle bender splint
    B. De Quervains splint
    C. Cock-up splint
    D. Posterior tube splint
24. What kind of orthosis is given in genu recurvatum?
    A. Recurvatum boots   B. KAFO
    C. HKAFO   D. All of the above
25. In a patient no power in ankle dorsi flexors, and with normal hip and knee power what kind of orthosis is given?
    A. Above knee orthosis
    B. AFO with foot drop stop
    C. Knee cage orthosis
    D. AFO, ankle joint in dorsiflexion stop
26. What will be the resultant force at the knee of a child having spasticity of plantar flexors attempting to walk plantigrade:
    A. Knee flexion   B. Knee rotation
    C. Knee extension   D. None of the above

20. A   21. D   22. B   23. B   24. B   25. B   26. C

Section II: Therapeutic Management

27. **Aeroplane splint is given with shoulder joint:**
    A. Extended
    B. Adducted
    C. Flexed
    D. Abducted
28. **Thoracolumbosacral orthosis is given for following conditions, *except*:**
    A. Vertebral compression fracture
    B. Intervertebral disc diseases
    C. Nonoperative and postoperative immobilization of spine
    D. Pelvic fractures
29. **Type of orthosis used to provide contralateral hip extension with ipsilateral hip flexion:**
    A. Pavlik harness
    B. Swivel orthosis
    C. Reciprocating gait orthosis
    D. None of the above
30. **Knuckle bender splint is given when there is:**
    A. Radial nerve injury
    B. Ulnar nerve injury
    C. Median nerve injury
    D. All of the above
31. **Following are considerations while selecting the footwear for a diabetic patient, *except*:**
    A. Comfort
    B. Distribution of forces over sufficiently large surface area
    C. Foot completely closed inside shoe, with a narrow ball
    D. Relief of pressure at sensitive areas
32. **The instruction in prescribing calipers:**
    A. Allow joint movements whenever possible and appropriate
    B. Orthosis should be functional throughout all phases of gait
    C. Static and dynamic alignment must be checked before giving the caliper to the patient
    D. All of the above
33. **What kind of modification to the shoe should be given to a patient having osteoarthritis of the medial compartment of the knee?**
    A. Thomas heel
    B. Lateral wedge insole
    C. Heel cushion
    D. Metatarsal bar

27. D   28. D   29. C   30. B   31. C   32. D   33. B

34. For plantar fasciitis with calcaneal spur, what kind of modification to the shoe should be given from the following?
    A. Heel cushion with microcellular rubber insole
    B. Metatarsal pad or bars
    C. High quarter shoes
    D. High heels
35. The splint given for patients with C6 complete tetraplegia?
    A. Knuckle bender splint
    B. Aeroplane splint
    C. Tenodesis splint
    D. None

34. A   35. C

CHAPTER 13

Prosthetics

1. **What do you mean by myoplasty with reference to amputation?**
   A. Attachment of anterior and posterior compartment muscles to each other over the end of the bone
   B. An artificial insertion is made by drilling a hole in a bone and insertion point is covered by periosteum
   C. An artificial insertion is made by drilling a hole in a bone and periosteum is stripped
   D. None of the above
2. **Absence of all four limbs is referred to as:**
   A. Transverse hemimelia
   B. Tetra-amelia
   C. Longitudinal hemimelia
   D. Phocomelia
3. **The range of supination and pronation in a below elbow (BE) amputation decreases as:**
   A. The length of below elbow stump increases
   B. The length of below elbow stump decreases
   C. The patient grows older
   D. The prosthesis is fitted with an artificial elbow joint
4. **Amputation through the elbow joint is referred to as:**
   A. Transhumeral amputation
   B. Elbow disarticulation
   C. Below elbow amputation
   D. Krukenberg amputation

1. A   2. B   3. B   4. B

5. **Splitting BE stump longitudinally at the interosseous membrane into radial and ulnar rays is referred to as:**
   A. Krukenberg amputation
   B. Below elbow amputation
   C. Wrist disarticulation
   D. Wallenberg's amputation
6. **External hemipelvectomy is also known as:**
   A. Hind quarter amputation
   B. Fore quarter amputation
   C. Hip disarticulation only
   D. Removal of pelvic bones only
7. **Lisfranc amputation is at the level of:**
   A. Forefoot
   B. Tarsometatarsal joint
   C. Metatarsophalangeal joints
   D. Ankle
8. **Functional upper extremity mechanical prosthesis is more effective in:**
   A. Above elbow amputation
   B. Forequarter amputation
   C. Below elbow amputation
   D. Elbow disarticulation
9. **Endoskeletal prosthesis works on the basis of:**
   A. Outer laminated shell weight bearing
   B. Internal modular components and tubing bearing weight
   C. Cosmesis alone
   D. Principle of Jordan
10. **Suspension for upper limb prosthesis is:**
    A. Silesian bandage
    B. Figure-of-eight harness
    C. Clavicular cuff
    D. Supracondylar cuff
11. **Muenster type of socket is used for:**
    A. Above elbow stump
    B. Very short upper extremity stump
    C. Wrist disarticulation
    D. Shoulder disarticulation

5. A   6. A   7. B   8. C   9. B   10. B   11. B

Section II: Therapeutic Management

12. The solid ankle cushion heel provides:
    A. Limited dorsiflexion and plantar flexion of foot
    B. No dorsiflexion, inversion or eversion
    C. Minimal inversion and eversion
    D. None of the above
13. What type of prosthesis will provide full weight bearing at end of stump?
    A. Conventional Syme's prosthesis
    B. PTB prosthesis
    C. Muensters prosthesis
    D. AK prosthesis
14. What type of prosthesis is given to the patient with bilateral transfemoral amputation?
    A. Syme's prosthesis   B. Bilateral below knee prosthesis
    C. Stubby prosthesis   D. None of the above
15. Syme's amputation is at:
    A. Transfemoral level
    B. Transtibial level
    C. Foot removed but heel pad preserved
    D. Metatarsophalangeal level
16. For a below knee amputation you should:
    A. Keep a pillow under the knee
    B. Place the stump over the opposite lower limb
    C. Keep the knee in flexed position in long sitting
    D. Keep the knee in extended position while sitting
17. The following prosthesis needs an elbow joint:
    A. Wrist disarticulation prosthesis
    B. Elbow disarticulation prosthesis
    C. Below elbow prosthesis
    D. Myoelectric hand
18. If a patient has to use more than one terminal device, the wrist joint commonly used is the:
    A. Flexion wrist unit
    B. Standard friction wrist unit
    C. Quick disconnect wrist unit
    D. Dorrance wrist unit

12. B   13. A   14. C   15. C   16. D   17. B   18. C

19. The features of myoelectric prosthesis are the following, *except*:
    A. Contraction of extensor muscle group of the residual stump opens the terminal device
    B. Controls fine motor rhythmic fast movements
    C. Uses normal muscle stimuli
    D. Less energy expenditure than mechanical prosthesis
20. The foot that cannot be cosmetically used by the amputee inside temple is:
    A. SACH foot
    B. Jaipur foot
    C. Madras foot
    D. None of the above
21. The thickest wall in quadrilateral socket is:
    A. Medial   B. Lateral
    C. Posterior   D. Anterior
22. Most energy expenditure in upper extremity prosthetics is in the use of:
    A. Voluntary closing hand
    B. Cosmetic hand
    C. Voluntary opening hand
    D. All of the above
23. The full form of SACH is:
    A. Standard active cushioned heel
    B. Solid ankle constructed heel
    C. Standard ankle cushion heel
    D. Solid ankle cushioned heel
24. The Bowden's dual control cable system operates:
    A. The shoulder joint and the wrist joint
    B. The elbow joint and the wrist joint
    C. The elbow joint and the terminal device
    D. The wrist joint and the terminal device
25. Soft inserts are given in the socket for amputees with the following conditions, *except*:
    A. Hansen's disease
    B. Diabetic sensory neuropathy
    C. Loss of sensation over the stump
    D. None of the above

19. B   20. A   21. C   22. A   23. D   24. C   25. D

Section II: Therapeutic Management

26. The most common amputation seen among lower extremity amputees due to dysvascular causes is:
    A. Transfemoral
    B. Syme's
    C. Toe amputation
    D. Transtibial amputation
27. When the lower limb is amputated below knee, the standard transtibial amputation is approximately what percentage of the tibial length?
    A. <10
    B. 20–50
    C. >70
    D. >80
28. Maximum energy expenditure is seen in:
    A. Unilateral BK prosthetic use
    B. Hip disarticulation prosthetic use
    C. Unilateral AK prosthetic use
    D. Syme's prosthetic use

26. C   27. B   28. B

CHAPTER 14

Mobility Aids

1. **If the patient needs a walking stick due to osteoarthritis of the hip on one side, on which side should he hold the stick?**
   A. The side of normal lower extremity
   B. The affected side of lower extremity
   C. Depends on his convenience
   D. Depends on the positive supporting reaction
2. **The crutch where measurement is taken from the olecranon with the elbow flexed to 90°:**
   A. Axillary crutch   B. Elbow crutch
   C. Gutter crutch   D. Tripod crutch
3. **Which muscles are needed for use of axillary crutches?**
   A. Depressors and adductors of the shoulder girdle, flexors of shoulder, extensors of elbow, dorsiflexors of the wrist
   B. Depressors and adductors of the shoulder girdle, flexors of shoulder, flexors of elbow, dorsiflexors of wrist
   C. Elevators and abductors of the shoulder girdle, extensors of shoulder, flexors of elbow, palmar flexors of wrist
   D. Elevators and abductors of the shoulder girdle, extensors of shoulder, flexors of elbow, palmar flexors of wrist
4. **To prevent equinus what modification in the wheelchair should be given from the following?**
   A. Avoid a foot rest
   B. Foot rest angled at 90°
   C. Foot straps
   D. Functional electrical stimulation

1. A   2. C   3. A   4. B

Section II: Therapeutic Management

5. Dependent transfers may be accomplished with a:
   A. Hoist
   B. Transfer board
   C. Hydraulic lift
   D. All of the above
6. The tip of the crutch, which is in contact with the ground, is called:
   A. Shoe
   B. PVC stub
   C. Ferrule
   D. Cane tip
7. The mobility aid from the list below which gives maximum stability is:
   A. Elbow crutch
   B. Walking stick
   C. Walking frame (walker)
   D. Axillary crutch
8. A person holding a white cane with a red tip indicates:
   A. He is hard of hearing
   B. The person has poor coordination
   C. Visual impairment
   D. Geriatric age group
9. Pneumatic tyres are ideally used in:
   A. Rough terrain
   B. Homes
   C. Offices
   D. Rest rooms
10. The following are controls of motorized wheelchairs, *except*:
    A. Joystick
    B. Hand rims
    C. Voice
    D. Puff of breath
11. Measurement of seat of wheelchair includes all the following, *except*:
    A. Width
    B. Height
    C. Cross sectional diameter
    D. Depth

5. D   6. C   7. C   8. C   9. A   10. B   11. C

12. The following are adaptations to the wheelchair, *except*:
    A. Light weight sports
    B. Motorization
    C. Brakes
    D. One arm drive
13. Paraplegic patients with pressure sores will need the following seat:
    A. Wooden
    B. Steel with padding around the edges
    C. Plastic
    D. Contoured foam
14. One of the following assistive devices is most appropriate initially for a patient with Parkinson's disease?
    A. Walker
    B. Rollator
    C. Axillary crutches
    D. Stable quadripod
15. The height of the grip of the walker should be taken from which anatomic stand point (patient in standing position)?
    A. Ulnar styloid process with elbow in flexed position
    B. Upper rim of Iliac crest
    C. 6 inches from the axilla
    D. Greater trochanter
16. Which anatomic structure should be used as a reference point in order to determine the proper backrest height for a standard wheelchair?
    A. Acromion   B. Scapula tip
    C. D11 spine   D. Costal margin
17. Forearm crutches or elbow crutches are also known as:
    A. Lofstrand crutches   B. Bernard's crutches
    C. Leonards crutches   D. Army crutches
18. A crutch has _____ points of contact with the body:
    A. 1
    B. 2
    C. 3
    D. Depends on the grip pattern

12. C   13. D   14. B   15. D   16. B   17. A   18. B

Section II: Therapeutic Management

19. The distance from the rubber ferrule laterally to the fifth toe (when measuring crutch length from the anterior axillary fold to the ground) is ____ inches.
    A. 2 inches
    B. 4 inches
    C. 6 inches
    D. 8 inches
20. A cane is prescribed in order to:
    A. Provide safety in balance disorders
    B. Reduce pathological pain
    C. Amplify proprioception
    D. All of the above
21. The anti tip bar is:
    A. A bar placed in front of the walker so that the person does not fall forward
    B. A bar in the sides of the rest room to prevent the person from falling
    C. A bar for disabled persons where employees do not accept tips
    D. A bar behind the wheelchair to prevent backward falls
22. A wheelchair which is propelled manually only by one hand is known as:
    A. Tetraplegic wheelchair
    B. Hemiplegic wheelchair
    C. Amputee wheelchair
    D. None of the above
23. Which of the following statements is false about wheelies?
    A. Is a maneuver in which a wheelchair is momentarily balanced on its rear wheel or wheels
    B. Needs training and practice
    C. Is used to clear small unevenness in the ground
    D. It is a safe maneuver
24. The following sport can be performed on a wheelchair?
    A. Chess
    B. Mountain biking
    C. Water skiing
    D. All of the above

19. C   20. D   21. D   22. B   23. D   24. D

CHAPTER 15

Vocational Rehabilitation

1. **Aptitude is:**
   A. The ability to perform ADL's independently
   B. The training given to a person so that he or she can be useful to society
   C. The absence of any mental abnormality which would normally hinder training
   D. Natural ability or talent in a special area
2. **Vocational rehabilitation is described as:**
   A. A process that assists individuals with impairments to overcome their handicaps and try to reintegrate them into society into a job
   B. Adaptation or adjustment of a patient to the impairment
   C. Rendering services to the patient in the community
   D. Motivating the family members to take care of the patient
3. **A disabled person put in a vocation should:**
   A. Not be a hazard to himself or others
   B. Be segregated
   C. Be treated with sympathy
   D. Inform all coworkers about his disability
4. **A person with residual poliomyelitis applying for a job and working alongside nondisabled persons is an example of:**
   A. Sheltered workshop
   B. Open employment
   C. Cooperatives
   D. Home-based employment

1. D   2. A   3. A   4. B

Section II: Therapeutic Management

5. The following model of vocational rehabilitation is most suitable for a quadriplegic:
   A. Home based
   B. Cooperative
   C. Sheltered workshop
   D. Open employment
6. The vocational counselor's duties are all of the following, *except*:
   A. Decision maker of the patient's vocation
   B. Arrange for the client to obtain direct experience of the working environment
   C. Evaluate interest aptitude and skill
   D. Ensure that the client has clear grasp of career structure
7. Reservation in government posts for the handicapped is an example of:
   A. Sheltered workshop
   B. Cooperative
   C. Open employment
   D. Self-employment
8. The employer of a disabled employee should:
   A. Earmark "light jobs" for him
   B. Allow him to work on the job without detailed job trial so that he does not feel discriminated
   C. Be given all his medical, family and personal details to enable efficient working
   D. None of the above
9. Groups of disabled people work in:
   A. Sheltered workshop   B. Self-employment
   C. Open employment   D. Home-based employment
10. Skill is:
    A. Talent that is inherited from ones parents
    B. Inherent capacity to perform ones activities of daily living
    C. An achieved level of performance resulting from training or practice
    D. None of the above

5. A   6. A   7. C   8. D   9. A   10. C

11. **Which of the following statements is true?**
    A. Skill training and aptitude have no correlation with one another
    B. If a person has good skill it means he does not need, or has not undergone training
    C. If a person has good aptitude, the effort to train his or her skill is reduced
    D. To be trained in a skill you need to be exceptionally intelligent
12. **Disabled persons can contribute to the country's economy if they properly fulfil the following criteria, *except* if:**
    A. They have the right skills
    B. They are placed in the right jobs
    C. They are given appropriate support where required
    D. They are ambulant
13. **Testing the capacity of skilled disabled job-seekers to hold down jobs in the open labour market is done through:**
    A. Scholarship schemes
    B. Job trials or work trials
    C. Skill training
    D. Incentives to the employers
14. **The purpose of job analysis is all of these, *except*:**
    A. To assess which jobs could be done by disabled persons if there is a future vacancy
    B. Whether the job or the working environment can be modified in some way to enable it to be done by disabled persons
    C. Which is the easiest job available that could be given to a disabled person
    D. If a job restructuring was to take place, which parts of a job could be done by a disabled person
15. **As per the order of the Indian Government it has been decided to extend the age concession of____years in favor of handicapped persons to recruitment to posts filled through the SSC and through Employment Exchange in Grade 'C' and Grade 'D' posts**
    A. 5 years   B. 10 years
    C. 15 years   D. No concession

11. C   12. D   13. B   14. C   15. B

Section II: Therapeutic Management

16. Each year on the occasion of the World Disabled Day, National Awards are given by the President of India to the following, *except*:
    A. Best employer of handicapped
    B. Best handicapped employee
    C. Best placement officer
    D. Highest profitability by an enterprise employing the disabled
17. Under the 'Scheme of Public Sector Banks for Orphanages, Women's Homes and Physically Handicapped Person', physically handicapped persons are eligible to take loans under the scheme, if they satisfy the following conditions, *except*:
    A. Should be pursuing a gainful occupation
    B. Family income from all sources should not exceed ₹ 7,200- p.a. in urban or semiurban areas
    C. Should prove that he or she is unemployed
    D. Should not have land holding exceeding 1 acre if irrigated, and 25 acres if unirrigated
18. Vocational rehabilitation consists of:
    A. Placing the individual back with a previous employer if a suitable position is available
    B. Evaluating the premorbid skills of a patient to see if an appropriate position exists
    C. Vocational testing
    D. All of the above
19. Factors preventing vocational rehabilitation include:
    A. Fear among the persons with disability, that cash payments and health benefits may be affected
    B. Views in society that disabled individuals cannot be as productive as 'normal' persons
    C. Employers' feelings that the disabled need to be employed out of 'sympathy'
    D. All of the above

16. D   17. C   18. D   19. D

CHAPTER 16

Pain and Musculoskeletal Disorders

1. Small myelinated fibers transmitting pricking pain are:
   A. A delta fibers
   B. C fibers
   C. A beta
   D. B fibers
2. Thalamic pain is usually concentrated in:
   A. Contralateral extremities
   B. Ipsilateral extremities
   C. Lower extremities
   D. Upper extremities
3. Gate control theory was proposed by:
   A. Goldscheider and Gelhard
   B. Von Frey
   C. Melzack and Wall
   D. Maveric and Walker
4. According to the Gate control theory of pain, stimulation of which fibers close the gate:
   A. Large diameter A beta fibers
   B. Small diameter A delta fibers
   C. C fibers
   D. All of the above
5. Risk factors for adhesive capsulitis (frozen shoulder) include all, *except*:
   A. Diabetes
   B. Pregnancy
   C. Hypothyroidism
   D. Stroke

1. A   2. A   3. C   4. A   5. B

Section II: Therapeutic Management

6. Gout is caused by deposits of crystals of _____ in the joint:
   A. Oxalate
   B. Stearate
   C. Urate
   D. Citrate

7. Which of the following is true about Mallet finger:
   A. It is a rupture of the terminal flexor tendon of the distal phalanx
   B. It is a rupture of the proximal extensor tendon of the proximal phalanx
   C. It is a rupture of the terminal extensor tendon of the distal phalanx
   D. It is a rupture of the proximal flexor tendon of the proximal phalanx

8. A chronic nontraumatic over use injury of the ulnar collateral ligament of the metacarpophalangeal (MCP) joint of the thumb is called:
   A. Boutonniere thumb
   B. Blackberry thumb
   C. Z thumb
   D. Gamekeepers thumb

9. Scheuermann's disease affects the:
   A. Hip
   B. Ankle
   C. Elbow joint
   D. Spine

10. The following is not an example of osteochondrosis:
    A. Sever's disease
    B. Osteogenesis imperfecta
    C. Kohler's disease
    D. Legg-Calve-Perthes disease

11. One of these muscles does not form part of the rotator cuff:
    A. Teres minor
    B. Teres major
    C. Infraspinatus
    D. Subscapularis

12. Writer's cramp:
    A. Affects the person only while writing
    B. Is due to local ischemia
    C. Will resolve with suitable antioxidants and vitamin E
    D. Is an activity specific focal dystonia

6. C   7. C   8. D   9. D   10. B   11. B   12. D

Chapter 16: Pain and Musculoskeletal Disorders

13. **Myositis ossificans is:**
    A. An inflammation of muscle
    B. Often happens without trauma
    C. A form of heterotopic ossification
    D. A hereditary disease
14. **All the following about Osgood Schlatter's disease are true, *except*:**
    A. It is a traction apophysitis
    B. It can cause pain and swelling below the knee joint anteriorly
    C. The common age group is 60 and above
    D. Games like basket ball can aggravate the pain
15. **Endorphins are chemicals that:**
    A. Are prescribed for pain relief
    B. Act similar to opioids
    C. Are reduced during physical activity
    D. Induce suicidal tendencies
16. **The ulnar nerve innervates which of these muscles:**
    A. Extensor carpi ulnaris
    B. Abductor pollicis longus
    C. Abductor pollicis brevis
    D. Abductor digiti minimi
17. **A Bankart lesion is:**
    A. Injury of the anteroinferior aspect of the glenoid labrum
    B. Injury of the superolateral aspect of the glenoid labrum
    C. Typically associated with a posterior dislocation of the shoulder
    D. A chip fracture of the humerus in the subacromial region
18. **The common radiological finding with Sudeck's atrophy or CRPS is:**
    A. Heterotopic bone formation
    B. Joint spaces obliterated
    C. Patchy osteopenia
    D. Schmorl's nodes
19. **Kienbock's disease is avascular necrosis of the:**
    A. Scaphoid
    B. Triquetrum
    C. Lunate
    D. Capitate

13. C   14. C   15. B   16. D   17. A   18. C   19. C

Section II: Therapeutic Management

20. Primary hyperuricaemia is due to increased ____ in the diet:
    A. Glycine
    B. Purine
    C. Alanine
    D. None of the above
21. A prolapsed disc is due to protrusion of:
    A. Entire intervertebral disc
    B. Nucleus pulposus
    C. Annulus fibrosus
    D. All of the above
22. In Dupuytren's contracture there is thickening and shortening of:
    A. Palmar fascia
    B. Superficial flexor tendons
    C. Deep flexor tendons
    D. All of the above
23. Tennis elbow:
    A. Is a lesion of the common flexor tendon
    B. Presents with pain and tenderness over the lateral epicondyle
    C. Does not affect grip strength
    D. Is diagnosed by X-ray of elbow joint
24. Which of the following provocative tests is specific for biceps tendonitis?
    A. Hawkins' test
    B. Neer's test
    C. Speed's test
    D. Empty can test
25. Which splint is used for De Quervain's tenosynovitis?
    A. Knuckle bender splint
    B. Thumb spica splint
    C. Cock up splint
    D. Frog splint
26. Which of the following regarding Adson's test is true?
    A. Used to detect thoracic outlet syndrome
    B. Used to rule out Erb's palsy
    C. Useful in detecting carpal tunnel syndrome
    D. Used to detect median nerve injury

20. B   21. B   22. A   23. B   24. C   25. B   26. A

CHAPTER 17

Surgery in Rehabilitation

1. **Causes for development of secondary deformity are the following, *except*:**
   A. Hypotonicity
   B. Hypertonicity
   C. Improper posture
   D. Early primi
2. **A cochlear implant is a device that:**
   A. Has a single component amplifying the input signal
   B. Is implanted under local anesthesia
   C. Stimulates the auditory nerve
   D. Stimulates the tympanic membrane
3. **The Ilizarov technique is used in all these conditions, *except*:**
   A. Fixed flexion deformities of the knee
   B. Shoulder dislocation
   C. Shortened limb for limb lengthening
   D. Scoliosis
4. **One of the techniques for Achilles tendon lengthening is:**
   A. Y-plasty
   B. T-plasty
   C. Modified T-plasty
   D. Z-plasty
5. **Eggers procedure is used for contracture of the:**
   A. Knee
   B. Hip
   C. Ankle
   D. Sternocleidomastoid

1. D   2. C   3. B   4. D   5. A

Section II: Therapeutic Management

6. Dr Paul Brand is well known for his surgical procedures in the management of:
   A. Filariasis
   B. Fractures
   C. Hansen's disease
   D. Myositis ossificans
7. Brand's four tailed procedure uses:
   A. Flexor to extensor tendon transfer
   B. Extensor carpi radialis longus tendon as donor
   C. Flexor carpi radialis tendon as donor
   D. All of the above
8. The principles of tendon transfer surgery are all, *except*:
   A. Donor muscle must be expendable
   B. Donor muscle should have a similar excursion to the tendon being replaced
   C. Donor muscle must be of adequate length
   D. Donor muscle power must be minimum 2 in MRC grading
9. Which of the following is useful in training the transferred tendon after surgery?
   A. Constraint-induced movement therapy
   B. Biofeedback
   C. Acupuncture
   D. Ultrasound massage
10. Surgery in the following condition is avoided through the Ponseti method:
    A. Knee flexor tightness
    B. Pressure sores
    C. Bilateral adductor tightness
    D. Congenital talipes equino varus (CTEV)
11. The stage in which the epidermis breaks down in a pressure sore is:
    A. Stage 1
    B. Stage 2
    C. Stage 3
    D. Stage 4

6. C   7. B   8. D   9. B   10. D   11. B

Chapter 17: Surgery in Rehabilitation

12. **Surgery is usually not indicated in the following stage of the pressure sore:**
    A. Stage 4
    B. Stage 3
    C. Stage 2
    D. Stage 5
13. **Metastasis in the spine is more common in the:**
    A. Sacral region
    B. Cervical region
    C. Lumbar region
    D. Thoracic region
14. **Surgical intervention is required in which nerve injury?**
    A. Sunderland degree 5
    B. Sunderland degree 6
    C. Sunderland degree 1
    D. Sunderland degree 2
15. **Surgery done in spinal canal stenosis:**
    A. JESS
    B. Ilizarov fixation
    C. Luque rod fixation
    D. Laminectomy
16. **Harrington rod is used to correct deformities of the:**
    A. Tibia
    B. Femur
    C. Spine
    D. Humerus
17. **The Younts procedure is the release of:**
    A. Tendoachilles
    B. Iliotibial (IT) band
    C. Adductor tendons
    D. Biceps tendon
18. **The intrathecal baclofen pump that is surgically implanted, is used to treat:**
    A. Intractable pain
    B. Contractures
    C. Incoordination
    D. Spasticity

12. C　13. D　14. A　15. D　16. C　17. B　18. D

Section II: Therapeutic Management

19. Metabolic changes that are found in patients with spinal cord injury that predispose to stone formation, are all, *except*:
    A. Increased urinary calcium
    B. Reduced urinary citrate
    C. Increased urinary specific gravity
    D. Increased hydration
20. In a patient with scoliosis, surgery is usually indicated if the Cobb's angle is greater than:
    A. 20°
    B. 40°
    C. 10°
    D. 30°
21. Craniotomy is done for all of the following, *except*:
    A. Traumatic epidural hematoma
    B. Subdural hematoma
    C. Increased intracranial pressure
    D. Severe migraine
22. Rehabilitation surgeries done in patients with cerebral palsy include all of the following, *except*:
    A. Hamstring fractional lengthening
    B. TA lengthening
    C. Adductor tenotomy
    D. Laminectomies

19. D   20. B   21. D   22. D

CHAPTER 18

Physical Agents

1. Following are indications to ice treatment, *except*:
   A. Pain and muscle spasm
   B. Acute inflammation following trauma
   C. Spasticity
   D. Peripheral occlusive vascular disease
2. Indications for paraffin wax therapy are all of the following, *except*:
   A. Pain and muscle spasm
   B. Adhesion and scar
   C. Rheumatoid arthritis
   D. Impaired skin sensation
3. The type of LASER used to treat musculoskeletal pain is:
   A. Gas dynamic LASER
   B. Helium silver LASER
   C. Helium mercury LASER
   D. Low level LASER
4. Contraindications to SWD include the following, *except*:
   A. Malignancy
   B. Pace makers
   C. Recent radiotherapy
   D. Nonsteroidal anti-inflammatory drugs (NSAIDs)
5. Traction force in intermittent cervical traction is:
   A. 7-10% body weight
   B. 1-2% of the body weight
   C. 1/3rd of the body weight
   D. None of the above

1. D   2. D   3. D   4. D   5. A

Section II: Therapeutic Management

6. In case of acute injury the following are done, *except*:
   A. Rest
   B. Wax bath
   C. Elevation
   D. Ice
7. Causalgia and sympathetic dystrophy pain in the upper limb can be treated by:
   A. Iontophoresis
   B. Interferential therapy (IFT)
   C. Surgery to the fingers
   D. Cryotherapy
8. Therapeutic effects of hydrotherapy include the following, *except*:
   A. Relief of pain and muscle spasm
   B. Improvement of circulation
   C. Functional activities restoration
   D. Reduction in tinnitus
9. The therapeutic effects of superficial heat include the following, *except*:
   A. Acceleration of healing
   B. Relief of spasm
   C. Acceleration of circulation
   D. Stimulation of hypothalamus
10. Physiological change due to heating is:
    A. Decreased metabolic rate
    B. Stimulation of sensory nerves
    C. Increased viscosity
    D. Decreased collagen extensibility
11. Minimal current required to produce a response with infinite duration of stimulus is referred to as:
    A. Chronaxie
    B. Rheobase
    C. Van Hoff point
    D. Lewis stimulation point
12. Which of the following is not a pure heating method?
    A. Wax bath
    B. Electric heating pads
    C. Contrast bath
    D. None of the above

6. B   7. B   8. D   9. D   10. B   11. B   12. C

Chapter 18: Physical Agents

13. The condensor field method for applying SWD includes these, *except*:
    A. Contraplanar
    B. Coplanar
    C. Crossfire
    D. Bipolar

14. The commonly used frequency of SWD is:
    A. 27.12 MHz
    B. 27.12 GHz
    C. 271.2 MHz
    D. 26.58 GHz

15. Possible complications of using direct current would be all of the below, *except*:
    A. Burns
    B. Current shock
    C. Skin irritation
    D. Increased sweating

16. The creation of an electromotive force (EMF) by way of a moving magnetic field around an electric conductor is:
    A. Electromagnetic induction
    B. Inductive reactance
    C. Eddy currents
    D. Transformer

17. The minimum time required for excitation of a neuron by a constant electric current of twice the threshold voltage:
    A. Rheobase
    B. Chronaxie
    C. Van Hoff point
    D. Lewis stimulation point

18. When the nerve adapts itself to a slowly increasing strength of stimulus the mechanism is known as:
    A. Depolarization
    B. Accommodation
    C. Iontophoresis
    D. Phonophoresis

13. D   14. A   15. D   16. A   17. B   18. B

Section II: Therapeutic Management

19. **Following are the electrodiagnostic tests to detect nerve lesions,** *except*:
    A. Nerve conduction velocity (NCV)
    B. Electromyography (EMG)
    C. Strength-duration (SD) curve
    D. Positron emission tomography (PET)

20. **Therapeutic effects of ultraviolet irradiation are as follows,** *except*:
    A. Formation of vitamin D
    B. Improved resistance to infection
    C. Pigmentation and improved condition of the skin
    D. Increased activity of sweat glands

21. **Contraindication to UV rays is as follows,** *except*:
    A. Pulmonary tuberculosis
    B. Acute eczema or dermatitis
    C. Acne vulgaris
    D. All the above

22. **LASER is used in the following conditions,** *except*:
    A. Ulcer over the skin
    B. Psoriasis
    C. Low back ache
    D. Metastatic bone disease

23. **Indication for interferential therapy include all of the following,** *except*:
    A. Brachialgia
    B. Back pain
    C. Rheumatic conditions
    D. Thrombophlebitis

24. **The concept of two medium frequency currents to produce a beat frequency effect within the body is used by:**
    A. LASER
    B. Interferential therapy (IFT)
    C. Transcutaneous electrical nerve stimulation (TENS)
    D. Short wave diathermy (SWD)

19. D   20. D   21. C   22. D   23. D   24. B

25. **Uses of TENS include all of the following, *except*:**
    A. Postherpetic neuralgia
    B. Causalgia
    C. Phantom pain
    D. Cardiac arrhythmias
26. **Reflex sympathetic dystrophy includes:**
    A. Shoulder hand syndrome
    B. Sudeck's atrophy
    C. Reflex neurovascular dystrophy
    D. All of the above
27. **A denervated muscle is stimulated by:**
    A. Galvanic current
    B. Faradic current
    C. Both of the above
    D. None of the above

25. D   26. D   27. A

III Management of Special Populations

SECTION OUTLINE

19. Hereditary and Congenital Problems
20. Ergonomics

CHAPTER 19

Hereditary and Congenital Problems

1. Neurofibromatosis is otherwise known as:
   A. Shy Drager syndrome
   B. Paget's diseases
   C. von Recklinghausen's disease
   D. Duchenne muscular dystrophy
2. Frequent fractures, blue sclera, deafness are seen in:
   A. Osteogenesis imperfecta
   B. Marfan's syndrome
   C. Ehler-Danlos syndrome
   D. Marble bone disease
3. Failure of segmentation of cervical vertebrae is known as:
   A. Klippel-Feil syndrome
   B. Sprengel's shoulder
   C. Arthrogryphosis
   D. Torticollis
4. Partial absence of at least one limb is known as:
   A. Meromelia
   B. Amelia
   C. Phocomelia
   D. Syringomelia
5. Which of these is not a congenital manifestation or birth defect?
   A. Sprengel shoulder
   B. Osteogenesis imperfecta
   C. Spina bifida
   D. Amyotropic lateral sclerosis

1. C   2. A   3. A   4. A   5. D

Section III: Management of Special Populations

6. Congenital torticollis is asymmetric deformity of neck due to contracture of:
   A. Trapezius
   B. Strenocleidomastoid
   C. Omohyoid
   D. Rhomboideus major
7. Trisomy 21 is seen in:
   A. Down's syndrome
   B. Duchenne muscular dystrophy
   C. Turner's syndrome
   D. Klinefelter's syndrome
8. Patella alta is when:
   A. The patella is absent
   B. The patella is fused with the femoral condyle
   C. The patella is placed low in relation to the knee joint
   D. The patella is placed high in relation to the knee joint
9. In Turner's syndrome, the genetic abnormality is in the chromosome:
   A. Y chromosome
   B. 22
   C. 24
   D. X chromosome
10. The components of club foot are all, *except*:
    A. Equinus
    B. Calcaneus
    C. Forefoot adductus
    D. Hindfoot varus
11. Morquio's syndrome is:
    A. X linked recessive   B. Y linked dominant
    C. X linked dominant   D. None of the above
12. One of these syndromes is not classified under the mucopolysaccharidoses:
    A. Hurler's syndrome
    B. San Filippo's syndrome
    C. Shy-dragers syndrome
    D. Hunter's syndrome

| 6. B | 7. A | 8. D | 9. D | 10. B | 11. D | 12. C |

Chapter 19: Hereditary and Congenital Problems

13. **Hypermobility of the joints is a feature of which syndrome?**
    A. Sjogren's syndrome
    B. Ehlers-Danlos syndrome
    C. Waardenburg syndrome
    D. All of the above

14. **All statements about Rett syndrome are true, *except*:**
    A. The disorder is almost always inherited from the mother
    B. The disorder is linked to the MECP 2 gene
    C. It almost always affects females
    D. The symptoms are due to mutation in the X chromosome

15. **Wilsons disease is a disease in which there is excess build up of:**
    A. Zinc
    B. Lipoprotein
    C. Copper
    D. Iron

16. **The genetic makeup of Klinefelter's syndrome is:**
    A. 47, XYY
    B. 46, XYY
    C. 46, XXY
    D. 47, XXY

17. **Tetralogy of Fallot is made of these components, except**
    A. Ventricular septal defect (VSD
    B. Overriding aorta
    C. Pulmonary artery stenosis
    D. Left ventricular hypertrophy

18. **Absence of proximal or middle segments of a limb with all or part of the distal segment present is called:**
    A. Transverse phocomelia
    B. Intermediate hemimelia
    C. Transverse intercalary limb deficiency
    D. Transverse integumental limb deficiency

19. **Werdnig Hoffman disease is a type of:**
    A. Motor neuron disease
    B. Sensory ataxia
    C. Cerebellopontine lesion
    D. Spinal muscular atrophy

13. B 14. A 15. C 16. D 17. D 18. C 19. D

Section III: Management of Special Populations

20. Urinary incontinence is a common symptom associated with all, *except*:
    A. Spina bifida
    B. Osteogenesis imperfecta
    C. Muscular dystrophy
    D. Down's syndrome

21. Complications of spina bifida may include all of the following, *except*:
    A. Charcot joints
    B. Pressure ulcers
    C. Neurogenic bladder
    D. Folic acid deficiency

22. All of the following may be associated with Arnold-Chiari malformation, *except*:
    A. Spina bifida cystica
    B. Myelomeningocele
    C. Spondylolisthesis
    D. Meningocele

23. Barlow and Ortolani tests done under ultrasound observation are helpful in detecting:
    A. Bilateral hip dislocation
    B. Congenital talipes equinovarus (CTEV)
    C. Spinal dysraphism
    D. Cerebral palsy

24. The following are types of hereditary motor sensory neuropathy, a group of inherited diseases of peripheral nerves affecting both motor and sensory nerves, *except*:
    A. Charcot-Marie Tooth disease
    B. Dejerine-Sottas disease
    C. Refsum's disease
    D. Werdnig-Hoffman disease

20. B   21. D   22. C   23. A   24. D

CHAPTER 20

Ergonomics

1. Synonyms for RSI (Repetitive strain injuries) include all, *except*:
   A. Musculoskeletal disorders (MSD)
   B. Cumulative trauma disorders (CTD)
   C. Occupational overuse syndrome (OOS)
   D. Repetitive neuromuscular disorders (RNMD)
2. The father of occupational health is:
   A. Dr Osler
   B. Dr Bernardino Rammazzini
   C. Dr Luciani
   D. Dr Lister
3. The compression at two or more locations along the course of a peripheral nerve is called:
   A. Double neurotmesis
   B. Dual paresthesia
   C. Double crush syndrome
   D. None of the above
4. Stenosing tenosynovitis in the fingers is also known as:
   A. Mallet finger
   B. Volkmann's contracture
   C. Trigger finger
   D. De Quervain's tenosynovitis
5. The maximum recommended load weight or load constant to be lifted under ideal conditions works out to:
   A. 41 pounds
   B. 45 pounds
   C. 59 pounds
   D. 51 pounds

1. D   2. B   3. C   4. C   5. D

6. The following task variables are measured with the person doing the job to calculate the recommended weight limit, *except*:
   A. Speed of activity
   B. Vertical travel distance
   C. Asymmetric angle
   D. Coupling
7. The tool(s) to assess musculoskeletal risk during a particular task for the entire body in standing posture:
   A. Rapid Upper Limb Assessment (RULA)
   B. Lifting index
   C. Rapid Entire Body Assessment (REBA)
   D. All of the above
8. While working at the computer workstation the monitor should be placed so that:
   A. The top of the screen should be slightly above the eye level
   B. The center of the screen should be at eye level
   C. The center of the screen should be slightly below eye level
   D. The top of the screen should be at or slightly below eye level
9. The distance from eyes to the monitor should be:
   A. 10–20 inches
   B. 18–30 inches
   C. 30–40 inches
   D. 24–40 inches
10. The very first ILO Convention adopted in 1919 fixes working time in industry with a few exceptions, to a maximum of:
    A. Nine hours per day with weekends off
    B. Eight hours per day with two days off per week
    C. Eight hours per day and 48 hours per week
    D. Eight hours per day and 40 hours per week
11. The curves in the spine are as follows:
    A. Cervical kyphosis, lumbar lordosis, thoracic kyphosis
    B. Cervical lordosis, thoracic kyphosis, lumbar kyphosis
    C. Cervical kyphosis, thoracic lordosis, lumbar lordosis
    D. Cervical lordosis, thoracic kyphosis, lumbar lordosis

6. A   7. C   8. D   9. B   10. C   11. D

Chapter 20: Ergonomics

12. **The Spurlings test for cervical radiculopathy is done by:**
    A. Simultaneous extension, rotation, lateral flexion of the neck away from the side of symptoms and vertical compression on the head
    B. Simultaneous flexion, rotation, lateral flexion of the neck away from the side of symptoms and vertical compression on the head
    C. Simultaneous extension, rotation, lateral flexion of the neck towards the side of symptoms and vertical compression on the head
    D. Simultaneous flexion, rotation, lateral flexion of the neck towards the side of symptoms and vertical compression on the head.
13. **The area that is easily reached with a sweep of the forearm across the workspace is called the:**
    A. Horizontal neutral inner reach zone
    B. Tertiary zone
    C. Secondary (outer reach zone)
    D. Working zone
14. **The lifting index (LI) is determined by the formula:**
    A. Recommended wight limit (RWL) ÷ Weight of the object lifted
    B. (Weight of the object actually lifted ÷ RWL) × 1/L1
    C. Weight of the object actually lifted ÷ RWL
    D. (Weight of the object actually lifted × RWL) ÷ Couplants
15. **The goal of ergonomic design is to have lifting jobs to accomplish a lifting index of:**
    A. >1 and <2 B. > or equal to 1
    C. <1   D. <0.5
16. **When assessing RULA scales, we must assess:**
    A. Both upper limbs at the same time
    B. Either of the upper limbs at any time and determine whether both UL need to be assessed
    C. Only the dominant upper limb
    D. Only one limb depending on which limb is used more
17. **For which REBA score will you implement change immediately because there is very high risk:**
    A. 7–9   B. 8–10
    C. >9   D. >11

12. C   13. A   14. C   15. C   16. B   17. D

IV Medical Conditions Needing Rehabilitation

SECTION OUTLINE

21. Burns
22. Brain Injury and Stroke
23. Lower Motor Neuron Lesions
24. Pediatric Rehabilitation and Cerebral Palsy
25. Orthopedics and Sports Rehabilitation
26. Diseases of the Muscle
27. Spinal Cord Injury
28. Movement Disorders
29. Cardiopulmonary Rehabilitation
30. Vascular and Hematological Conditions
31. Arthritis

CHAPTER 21

Burns

1. **One of the complications of improper splinting in burns with the limb kept in a comfortable position:**
   A. Abnormal pigmentation
   B. Dehydration
   C. Myopathy
   D. Contractures

2. **First-degree burns:**
   A. Are superficial burns involving only the epidermis
   B. Involve the whole depth of the dermis
   C. Involve a part of the dermis
   D. Involve a part of the dermis and epidermis

3. **Arrhythmias of the heart can be a result of:**
   A. Thermal burns
   B. Electrical burns
   C. Cold burns
   D. All of the above

4. **The least percentage in the rule of 9's is given to the following region:**
   A. Head
   B. Hand
   C. Genitals
   D. Lower back

5. **Destruction of melanocytes in burns can cause:**
   A. Contractures
   B. Ulcers
   C. Dark spots
   D. Hypopigmentation

1. D   2. A   3. B   4. C   5. D

Section IV: Medical Conditions Needing Rehabilitation

6. **What kind of physiotherapy is used to treat a patient with early burns who has not been skin grafted:**
   A. Passive movement of the joint perpendicular to the line of contraction of scar tissue
   B. No movement of the affected tissue
   C. Active movement against the line of contraction of scar tissue
   D. Active movement towards the line of contraction of scar tissue

7. **When a blister develops over a second-degree burn, we must:**
   A. Immediately remove the fluid inside with a sterile needle to prevent pus formation
   B. Immediately remove the fluid inside with a sterile needle so that dressing the wound is facilitated
   C. Avoid popping the blister
   D. Avoid popping the blister if the patient cannot bear the pain

8. **A patient is admitted in to hospital with severe burns. What complication do you have to, *expect*?**
   A. Hypovolemic shock
   B. Anemia
   C. Anaphylaxis
   D. Cardiogenic shock

9. **Perioral burns can result in:**
   A. Palatal palsy
   B. Aphasia
   C. Microstomia
   D. All of the above

10. **The Lund and Browder chart is used to assess:**
    A. The extent of splinting needed for the burn
    B. The extent of grafting needed for the burn
    C. The extent of rehabilitation needed for the victim
    D. The extent of burned body surface area in children

11. **Extremely hot environment should be avoided in patients with full thickness burns because:**
    A. It worsens hypertrophic scar formation
    B. Ability to cool the body through sweating is lost
    C. It worsens contracture formation
    D. All of the above

6. C   7. C   8. A   9. C   10. D   11. B

Chapter 21: Burns

12. The splint given to the hand to prevent a flexion (claw like) contracture in a palmar burn is a volar splint that keeps:
    A. The IP joints in extension, MCP in flexion, and the thumb in adduction
    B. The IP joints in flexion, MCP in flexion, and the thumb in 20° to 30° of abduction
    C. The IP joints in extension, MCP in flexion, and the thumb in 20–30° of abduction
    D. The IP joints in flexion, MCP in flexion, and the thumb in 20° to 30° of abduction
13. Psychological issue seen after burns:
    A. Post-traumatic stress disorder (PTSD)
    B. Adjustment disorders
    C. Depression
    D. All of the above
14. Second degree burns are also known as:
    A. First degree burns
    B. Full thickness burns
    C. Partial thickness burns
    D. Superficial burns
15. What percentage of total body surface area should be affected in order to classify as a major burn?
    A. Over 25%
    B. Over 40%
    C. Over 50%
    D. Over 90%
16. Airplane splints are fabricated to prevent contracture development after burns in which of the following areas:
    A. Neck
    B. Back
    C. Shoulder
    D. Groin
17. Pruritis (itch) is a significant complaint for many patients after burns. It is managed using all of the following, *except*:
    A. Passive stretching
    B. Topical moisturizer
    C. Oral gabapentin
    D. Transcutaneous electrical nerve stimulation (TENS)

12. C   13. D   14. C   15. A   16. C   17. A

Section IV: Medical Conditions Needing Rehabilitation

18. Debridement, which is the removal of eschar to expose viable tissue and prepare the wound bed for coverage consists of all of the following, *except*:
    A. Enzymatic debridement
    B. Mechanical debridement
    C. Immersion debridement
    D. Surgical debridement

19. Which of the following statements about splinting is not true:
    A. Used with patients who are not compliant with positioning
    B. Used if exposed tendons or joints are present.
    C. Splinting should be performed without mobilization
    D. Prevents contracture

20. Compression garments are used to help decrease:
    A. Pruritus
    B. Contracture
    C. Hypertrophic scarring
    D. Lymphatic flow

21. Most common site of heterotopic ossification involvement in burns is:
    A. Occipital protuberance
    B. Knee
    C. Elbow
    D. Wrist

18. C   19. C   20. C   21. C

CHAPTER 22

Brain Injury and Stroke

1. The Glasgow coma scale evaluates a patient according to all the following, *except*:
   A. Eye opening response
   B. Tendon reflexes
   C. Motor responses
   D. Verbal responses
2. Which of the following statements on constraint induced movement therapy is wrong?
   A. It is of use in patients with hemineglect
   B. The affected hand is constrained so that the normal hand is better used
   C. It is used in patients in whom there is some power and movement on the affected side
   D. None of the above
3. The following statements about TIA are true, *except*:
   A. They can serve as a warning for stroke
   B. The signs and symptoms resemble those of a stroke
   C. There is usually an acute infarction
   D. They do not last more than 24 hours
4. The most common cause of hemorrhagic stroke is:
   A. Aneurysms
   B. Head injury
   C. Bleeding disorders
   D. Uncontrolled hypertension

1. B   2. B   3. C   4. D

Section IV: Medical Conditions Needing Rehabilitation

5. The speech disorder commonly found in stroke is:
   A. Dysphonia
   B. Palatal dystonia
   C. Aphasia
   D. Sensory conduction dysphasia
6. Fluent speech is present in:
   A. Global aphasia
   B. Wernicke's aphasia
   C. Dysarthria
   D. None of the above
7. When a stroke patient denies ownership of body (for example of ones own limbs), it is called:
   A. Asomatognosia
   B. Anisognosia
   C. Hemineglect
   D. Denial
8. The three phases of swallowing include all, *except*:
   A. Pharyngeal
   B. Esophageal phases
   C. Glottal phase
   D. Oral phase
9. Cryptogenic stroke is:
   A. A stroke originating in the crypts of the brain
   B. A stroke without an identifiable cause
   C. A stroke where there is no evidence of an infarct
   D. A stroke affecting only the cranial nerves
10. The functions of the left brain are all the following, *except*:
    A. Logic
    B. Sequencing
    C. Calculation
    D. Intuition
11. Shoulder subluxation after stroke:
    A. More common in flaccid hemiplegia
    B. Is not influenced by spasticity
    C. Needs MRI scans for diagnosis
    D. Cannot be prevented

5. C   6. B   7. A   8. C   9. B   10. D   11. A

Chapter 22: Brain Injury and Stroke

12. The artery involved in lateral medullary syndrome is:
    A. Middle inferior cerebral
    B. Anterior superior cerebellar
    C. Posterior inferior cerebellar artery
    D. Posterior inferior cerebral artery
13. Inability to read is:
    A. Apraxia
    B. Acalculia
    C. Aphonia
    D. Alexia
14. The thrombolytic agent indicated for acute ischaemic stoke:
    A. Aldolase
    B. Heparin
    C. Alteplase
    D. Tryptase
15. The following statement about tissue plasminogen activator (tPA) is true:
    A. Can be given up to 24 hours after the onset of the stroke
    B. Causes breakdown of a clot by fibrinolysis
    C. Can be given in hemorrhagic stroke after taking bleeding and clotting time
    D. All of the above
16. Echolalia means:
    A. Trying to imitate another person's facial expressions
    B. Difficulty in expressing feelings
    C. Interspersing words with meaningless syllables
    D. Unsolicited repetition of another persons words
17. The artery most commonly involved in an epidural hematoma is the:
    A. Middle meningeal artery
    B. Posterior cerebral artery
    C. Vertebral artery
    D. Internal carotid artery
18. Decorticate rigidity has all the following components, *except*:
    A. Arms flexed, or bent inward on the chest
    B. The hands are clenched into fists
    C. Legs flexed with feet turned outward
    D. Legs extended and feet turned inward

12. C   13. D   14. C   15. B   16. D   17. A   18. C

19. What would a Glasgow coma scale range be:
    A. 3-15
    B. 0-15
    C. 1-15
    D. None of the above
20. Uncal herniation typically causes compression to the:
    A. Facial nerve
    B. Trigeminal nerve
    C. Occulomotor nerve
    D. Glossopharyngeal nerve
21. Spatial neglect is commonly seen in:
    A. Dominant hemisphere stroke
    B. Nondominant hemisphere stroke
    C. Brainstem strokes
    D. Cerebellar strokes
22. Excitotoxicity seen after traumatic brain injury is due to the release of which excitotoxic neurotransmitter:
    A. GABA
    B. Glutamate
    C. Dopamine
    D. Acetylcholine
23. Which of the statements about vegetative state is false?
    A. Absence of sleep-wake cycle on EEG
    B. No awareness of self or environment
    C. Presence of a verbal or auditory startle but no localization or tracking
    D. Patient opens eyes (either spontaneously or with noxious stimuli)
24. The term "permanent vegetative state" is used to denote irreversibility:
    A. After 6 months following nontraumatic brain injury and 18 months following traumatic brain injury
    B. After 12 months following nontraumatic brain injury and 3 months following traumatic brain injury
    C. After 3 months following nontraumatic brain injury and 12 months following traumatic brain injury
    D. After 18 months following nontraumatic brain injury and 6 months following traumatic brain injury

19. A   20. C   21. B   22. B   23. A   24. C

25. The disability rating scale evaluates all of the following, *except*:
    A. Feeding
    B. Toileting
    C. Grooming
    D. Stair climbing
26. According to Rancho Los Amigos levels of cognitive function scale, RLA 4 corresponds to:
    A. Localized response to stimuli
    B. Generalized response to stimulation
    C. Confused but appropriate behavior
    D. Confused and agitated behavior
27. Paroxysmal autonomic instability and dystonia (PAID) episodes seen after TBI consists of all of the following, *except*:
    A. Tachycardia
    B. Hyperthermia
    C. Vomiting
    D. Perspiration
28. The causes of hyponatremia associated with brain injury include all of the following, *except*:
    A. Syndrome of inappropriate antidiuretic hormone secretion (SIADH)
    B. Cerebral salt wasting
    C. Diabetes insipidus
    D. None of the above

25. D   26. D   27. C   28. C

CHAPTER 23

Lower Motor Neuron Lesions

1. **Which part of the body is commonly affected by the polio virus?**
   A. Brainstem and anterior horn cells of the spinal cord
   B. Cerebellum
   C. Hypothalamus
   D. Weakened muscles
2. **The final stage of poliomyelitis is the:**
   A. Infective stage
   B. Acute on chronic stage
   C. Residual stage
   D. Recovery stage
3. **The number of serotypes of poliovirus:**
   A. 4				B. 5
   C. 2				D. 3
4. **Which of the following statements about poliomyelitis is true?**
   A. In residual poliomyelitis there is always recovery in muscle power
   B. It never affects the muscles of breathing
   C. Upper limbs are affected more than the lower limbs
   D. None of the above
5. **The oral polio vaccine in use contains:**
   A. Inactivated virus
   B. Live attenuated virus
   C. Antibodies to poliovirus
   D. Killed polio microorganisms to the order of 10,000,000 organisms/mL

1. A   2. C   3. D   4. D   5. B

6. **The best antiviral agent for treating polio is:**
   A. Remdesivir
   B. Tocilizumab
   C. Azithromycin
   D. None of the above
7. **The MRC grading that is used to test muscle power in polio grades from:**
   A. 0–6
   B. 1–5
   C. 0–5
   D. All of the above
8. **Poliovirus is a type of:**
   A. Arbovirus
   B. Enterovirus
   C. Coronavirus
   D. Rotavirus
9. **Which of these organizations has partnered along with the World Health Organization in the Global Polio Eradication Initiative?**
   A. Rotary International
   B. The US Centers for Disease Prevention (CDC)
   C. The Bill and Melinda Gates Foundation
   D. All of the above
10. **As of October 2019 the following strains of wild polio have been eradicated:**
    A. Type 1 and 1
    B. Type 2 and 3
    C. Type 1 and 3
    D. Type 1 2 and 3
11. **The Halstead-Ross criteria for the diagnosis of post-polio syndrome consists of the following, *except*:**
    A. History of previous diagnosis of poliomyelitis
    B. Recovery of function with stability for about 15 years.
    C. Return of symptoms, usually because of a medical condition causing LMN weakness
    D. Fatigue and arthralgia causing difficulties in ADL's
12. **The angulation of deformities is measured by:**
    A. Manometer
    B. Angulometer
    C. Kinesiograph
    D. Goniometer

| 6. D | 7. C | 8. B | 9. D | 10. B | 11. C | 12. D |

Section IV: Medical Conditions Needing Rehabilitation

13. **Triple arthrodesis in polio involves fusion of:**
    A. Calcaneonavicular, calcaneocuboid, and talonavicular joints
    B. Talocalcaneal, calcaneocuboid, and talonavicular joints
    C. Talofibular, talocalcaneal and talonavicular joints
    D. Talofibular, talonavicular, and calcaneonavicular joints
14. **Muscle involvement in the lower limbs in polio is usually:**
    A. Symmetrical
    B. Confined to smaller muscles
    C. Proximal more than distal
    D. None of the above
15. **Loss of sensation in poliomyelitis:**
    A. Is due to Pacinian corpuscles involvement
    B. Is only in the cranial nerves
    C. Is due to corticospinal tract involvement
    D. Is very rare
16. **The inventor of the inactivated vaccine in polio was:**
    A. Dr Salk
    B. Dr Sabin
    C. Dr Alfred Williams
    D. All of the above
17. **Sister Kenny packs were used during the ____ phase of polio:**
    A. Post polio phase
    B. Acute phase
    C. Recovery phase
    D. Residual phase
18. **Which nerve is compressed in tarsal tunnel syndrome?**
    A. Posterior tibial nerve
    B. Lateral popliteal nerve
    C. Sural nerve
    D. Peroneal nerve
19. **The condition of the nerve where there is complete anatomical section (disruption) is known as:**
    A. Neuropraxia
    B. Axonotmesis
    C. Neurotmesis
    D. Complete nerve block

13. B   14. D   15. D   16. A   17. B   18. A   19. C

Chapter 23: Lower Motor Neuron Lesions

20. Common features seen in Bell's palsy include the following, *except*:
    A. Eye can be opened but cannot be closed
    B. The corner of mouth droops on affected side
    C. Food collects between teeth and cheek on the affected side
    D. Paralysis of the inferior rectus causing the eyeball to roll up

21. Care to be taken for eye of the patient suffering from Bell's palsy include these, *except*:
    A. To use glasses or goggles during the day
    B. To use moisturising ointment
    C. To advise the patient not to close the eyes too often
    D. To tape or patch the eyelids while asleep

22. Nerve conduction studies are helpful for diagnosis of:
    A. Efferent pathway lesion
    B. Afferent pathway lesion
    C. Both of above
    D. None of the above

23. The pronator syndrome is due to the compression of the:
    A. Median nerve
    B. Ulnar nerve
    C. Radial nerve
    D. Posterior interosseous nerve

24. 'Taking tip' attitude (adduction and internal rotation of shoulder, extended elbow, pronation of the forearm, and flexion of wrist) of limb indicates:
    A. Klumpke's palsy
    B. Thoracic outlet syndrome
    C. Erb's palsy
    D. Subscapularis contracture

25. Cubital tunnel syndrome refers to entrapment of:
    A. Ulnar nerve
    B. Median nerve
    C. Anterior interosseous nerve
    D. Radial nerve

26. **Klumpke's palsy involves:**
    A. C2 to C4
    B. C4 to C6
    C. C1 to C3
    D. C8 to T1

20. D   21. C   22. C   23. A   24. C   25. A   26. D

Section IV: Medical Conditions Needing Rehabilitation

27. **EMG is helpful in diagnosis of:**
    A. Denervation
    B. Renervation
    C. Myopathy
    D. All of the above
28. **The muscles paralyzed due to ulnar nerve injury below elbow, are all of the following, *except*:**
    A. Flexor carpi radialis
    B. Abductor digiti minimi
    C. Interossei
    D. Hypothenar muscles
29. **Which muscle causes compression of the median nerve?**
    A. Flexor carpi ulnaris
    B. Flexor digitorum profundus
    C. Pronator teres
    D. Pronator quadratus
30. **Deformity with hyperextension of the MCP joints and flexion of the IP joints (proximal and distal) is referred to as:**
    A. Claw hand deformity
    B. Wrist drop deformity
    C. Ape thumb deformity
    D. Pointing index deformity
31. **Wartenberg's syndrome is a specific mononeuropathy, caused by entrapment of the:**
    A. Inferior branch of the median nerve
    B. Superior branch of the ulnar nerve
    C. Superficial branch of the radial nerve
    D. Deep branch of the ulnar nerve
32. **F wave and H-reflex are seen on:**
    A. Electromyogram (EMG)
    B. Electroencephalogram (EEG)
    C. Nerve conduction velocity (NCV) test
    D. Ultrasonography (USG)

27. D   28. A   29. C   30. A   31. C   32. C

CHAPTER 24

Pediatric Rehabilitation and Cerebral Palsy

1. **The setting sun sign is seen in:**
   A. Hydrocephalus
   B. Osteogenesis imperfecta
   C. Spina bifida
   D. Microcephaly
2. **Most common risk factors for cerebral palsy is:**
   A. Prenatal risk factors
   B. Perinatal risk factors
   C. Postnatal risk factors
   D. Hereditary factors
3. **Damage to which part of brain causes athetosis?**
   A. Frontal lobe   B. Motor cortex
   C. Basal ganglia   D. Brainstem
4. **Obstructive hydrocephalus is commonly due to all, *except*:**
   A. Arnold-Chiari malformation
   B. Dandy-Walker malformation
   C. Aqueduct stenosis
   D. Wartenburg syndrome
5. **One of the following statements is not true about cerebral palsy:**
   A. There is motor disturbance especially in movement and posture
   B. Mental retardation may or may not be present
   C. Spastic cerebral palsy is the commonest
   D. The damage to the brain is progressive

1. A   2. A   3. C   4. D   5. D

Section IV: Medical Conditions Needing Rehabilitation

6. The oral antispasticity medication that works at the skeletal muscle level:
   A. Baclofen
   B. Diazepam
   C. Tizanidine
   D. Dantrolene

7. The incidence of neural tube defects (in the child) is reduced if one takes which vitamin (during pregnancy)?
   A. Thiamine
   B. Pyridoxine
   C. Folic acid
   D. Vitamin C

8. The following procedures can be done to treat spasticity, *except*:
   A. Injection of phenol
   B. Injection of botulinum toxin
   C. Intrathecal morphine
   D. Selective dorsal rhizotomy

9. Children with meningomyelocele (MMC) often present with the following conditions, *except*:
   A. Contractures of the upper limb
   B. Hydrocephalus
   C. Neurogenic bladder
   D. Precocious puberty

10. Most of the cases of cerebral palsy (CP) cases occur during which period?
    A. Neonatal
    B. Perinatal
    C. Infancy
    D. Prenatal

11. Cerebral palsy is defined as:
    A. A stroke in the young brain
    B. A disorder of movement control and posture resulting from a nonprogressive lesion in an immature brain.
    C. A damage to the brain of a child resulting in mental retardation
    D. A progressive lesion in the immature brain that affects the child continuously till he or she becomes an adult

6. D   7. C   8. C   9. A   10. D   11. B

Chapter 24: Pediatric Rehabilitation and Cerebral Palsy

12. When only one leg and one arm on the same side of the body in a child with cerebral palsy are involved it is called:
    A. Spastic diplegia
    B. Double hemiplegia
    C. Hemiplegia
    D. Triplegia
13. One of these conditions is a common cause of cerebral palsy
    A. Hypothyroidism in the child
    B. Frequent trauma to the head
    C. Trisomy 21
    D. Prematurity
14. Among the types of cerebral palsy which is the commonest?
    A. Mixed type
    B. Spastic
    C. Flaccid
    D. Choreoathetoid
15. Which milestone among these (at the age of about 2 years) is a good prognosticator for walking in the future?
    A. Social smile
    B. Segmental rolling
    C. Head and neck control
    D. Sitting independently
16. Between phenol and botulinum toxin in the management of spasticity in children with cerebral palsy, which of the following is false?
    A. Botulinum toxin is costlier than phenol
    B. Injection of phenol may cause irritation swelling and burning pain
    C. Botulinum toxin is longer lasting and has several side effects
    D. All of the above
17. What to do when the child has a seizure:
    A. Try to control the fit by restraining the extremities
    B. Force the mouth open and feed the child glucose to reduce violence of fits
    C. Lay the child supine in a calm place and gently leave
    D. None of the above
18. The surgery of adductor tenotomy should be considered:
    A. Only when the child has a dislocated hip and to prevent pain
    B. Only when the child attains bone maturity
    C. Only when scissoring prevents a good gait
    D. In severe spasticity as a means to prevent complications like dislocation of the hip

12. C   13. D   14. B   15. D   16. C   17. D   18. D

Section IV: Medical Conditions Needing Rehabilitation

19. The following is an indication for botulinum toxin in children:
    A. Congenital talipes equinovarus (CTEV)
    B. Ataxia
    C. Flexion contracture at the knee
    D. Focal dystonia
20. Physiotherapy may be started in children with cerebral palsy:
    A. When they achieve head and neck control
    B. When they are able to understand simple one stage commands
    C. When abnormal muscle tone exists and the diagnosis is not clear
    D. Once the MRI scans confirm the diagnosis
21. Intrathecal baclofen can be considered for:
    A. A child with knee flexion deformity and ankle deformity
    B. A child with Grade 1 spasticity
    C. A child with knee flexion deformity but no ankle deformity
    D. A child with Grade 3 spasticity or dystonia interfering with function and who has not responded to oral medications
22. Spastic cerebral diplegia means:
    A. The entire body is affected, including the trunk and all four extremities but the upper limbs are more involved
    B. Only the lower limbs are affected and the upper limbs are spared
    C. All four extremities are affected, but the legs are more affected than the arms or hands
    D. Only the muscles directly innervated by the cerebral cortex are spastic
23. The common pathognomonic lesion seen in cerebral palsy is:
    A. Hydrocephalus
    B. Periventricular leukomalacia (PVL)
    C. Arnold–Chiari malformation
    D. Temporal lobe infarct

19. D   20. C   21. D   22. C   23. B

CHAPTER
25
Orthopedics and Sports Rehabilitation

1. **In scoliosis, if the curve is greater than 60° then the following can be considered:**
   A. Exercise
   B. Milwaukee brace
   C. Surgery
   D. Psychological counseling
2. **Greenstick fractures occur mostly in:**
   A. Children
   B. Adolescents
   C. Old people
   D. All of the above
3. **Dinner fork deformity is seen in:**
   A. Colles' fracture
   B. Barton's fracture
   C. Smith's fracture
   D. Chauffeur's fracture
4. **Arthrodesis of knee may be indicated in the following, *except*:**
   A. Painful advanced OA or failed total knee replacements
   B. Acute septic arthritis
   C. Permanent correction of a deformity
   D. Gross knee instability in polio
5. **All are true for Sprengel's shoulder, *except*:**
   A. Scapula high in position
   B. Smaller scapula
   C. It is a congenital disorder
   D. Mostly normal shoulder movements

1. C   2. A   3. A   4. B   5. D

Section IV: Medical Conditions Needing Rehabilitation

6. Conditions predisposing to scoliosis can be due to all, *except*:
   A. Cerebral palsy
   B. Poliomyelitis
   C. Syringomyelia
   D. Gout
7. In complications of pediatric supracondylar fracture (extension type) the nerve most commonly injured is:
   A. Circumflex nerve
   B. Anterior interosseous nerve
   C. Ulnar nerve
   D. Brachial nerve
8. What happens to the lower limb in posterior hip dislocation?
   A. Flexed adducted and internally rotated
   B. Flexed abducted and internally rotated
   C. Flexed adducted and externally rotated
   D. Flexed abducted and externally rotated
9. A malignant tumor that produces osteoid:
   A. Chondroblastoma
   B. Chondrosarcoma
   C. Osteosarcoma
   D. Osteochondroma
10. A benign tumor in epiphysis is:
    A. Chondroblastoma
    B. Enchondroma
    C. Osteosarcoma
    D. Osteochondroma
11. Common type of elbow dislocation is:
    A. Anterior
    B. Posterior
    C. Medial
    D. Lateral
12. Medial apophysitis which occurs due to repetitive ball throwing in players is otherwise known as:
    A. Tennis elbow
    B. Golfer's elbow
    C. Little Leaguer's elbow
    D. Boxer's elbow

6. D   7. B   8. A   9. C   10. A   11. B   12. C

Chapter 25: Orthopedics and Sports Rehabilitation

13. **Galleazi fracture is:**
    A. Dislocation of radial head, with supracondylar fracture
    B. Dislocation of radial head with ulnar fracture
    C. Dislocation of distal radioulnar joint with fracture of the distal part of radius
    D. Fracture of the ulnar styloid

14. **_____ is inflammation at bony insertions of tendons, and ligaments:**
    A. Tendinitis
    B. Capsulitis
    C. Enthesitis
    D. All of the above

15. **Jones fracture is the:**
    A. Fracture of the fifth metatarsal
    B. Fracture of the lateral malleolus of the tibia
    C. Fracture of the medial malleolus of the tibia
    D. Fracture of the third metatarsal

16. **Guyon's canal is usually the site of entrapment of:**
    A. Radial nerve
    B. Median nerve
    C. Ulnar nerve
    D. Brachial nerve

17. **Which carpal bone is fractured most commonly?**
    A. Scaphoid
    B. Lunate
    C. Hamate
    D. Pisiform

18. **Severe radial club hand usually involves:**
    A. Absence of the thumb and ulna with radial deviation
    B. Absence of the thumb radius and carpal bones on the radial side with radial deviation
    C. Absence of the thumb and little finger with radial deviation of hand
    D. Absence of the thumb and radius with ulnar deviation of hand

19. **Tear drop fracture of the cervical spine is caused by:**
    A. Hyperflexion
    B. Hyperextension
    C. None of the above
    D. Both A and B

13. C   14. C   15. A   16. C   17. A   18. B   19. D

Section IV: Medical Conditions Needing Rehabilitation

20. The abnormality commonly associated with Klippel–Feil syndrome is:
    A. Scoliosis
    B. Bamboo spine
    C. Lordosis
    D. Arthrogryphosis

21. Slipping forward of one vertebra over the other is known as:
    A. Spondylolisthesis
    B. Spondylitis
    C. Spondylolysis
    D. Facetal joint dislocation

22. What is the common dislocation of the hip?
    A. Anterior
    B. Posterior
    C. Medial
    D. Lateral

23. A stress fracture of a metatarsal bone is:
    A. Boxer's fracture
    B. March fracture
    C. Bennet's fracture
    D. Barton's fracture

24. Hyperflexion of only the DIP joint of the toe is known as:
    A. Mallet toe
    B. Claw toe
    C. Hammer toe
    D. Bunion

25. Inflammation of the muscle tendon attachment caused by repeated strain on the attachment of the periosteum is known as:
    A. Bursitis
    B. Tendinitis
    C. Tenoperiostitis
    D. Tenosynovitis

26. Which ligament of the knee is commonly injured in sports?
    A. Anterior cruciate ligament (ACL)
    B. Posterior cruciate ligament (PCL)
    C. Both are equally injured
    D. None of the above

20. A   21. A   22. B   23. B   24. A   25. C   26. A

Chapter 25: Orthopedics and Sports Rehabilitation

27. **One of the clinical tests used to test meniscal tear is:**
    A. Schober's test
    B. McMurray's test
    C. Lachman's test
    D. Adsons test

28. **Apley's grind test is used to diagnose:**
    A. Meniscus tear
    B. Medial collateral ligament tear
    C. Posterior collateral ligament tear
    D. Anterior collateral ligament

29. **Which of the following statements is true:**
    A. Lachman's test is more sensitive than anterior drawer test
    B. Anterior drawer test is more sensitive than Lachman's test
    C. Lachman's test and anterior drawer test both are not sensitive
    D. All are false

30. **The treatment phases in sports rehabilitation include all of the following, *except*:**
    A. The first phase is to resolve the pain and inflammation
    B. The second phase is to restore ROM
    C. The third phase is strengthening
    D. The fourth phase is proprioceptive training and last phase involves sports or task specific activities
    E. None (all are true)

31. **The following statements are true about mallet finger, *except*:**
    A. A rupture of the terminal extensor tendon of the distal phalanx
    B. It is usually caused by forced flexion of the distal phalangeal joint
    C. It is usually caused by forced extension of the distal phalangeal joint
    D. Cricket and volley ball are common causes of mallet finger in our country.

32. **The specific training variable for an athlete includes:**
    A. Frequency of training
    B. Duration of training
    C. Intensity of training
    D. All of the above

27. B   28. A   29. A   30. E   31. C   32. D

Section IV: Medical Conditions Needing Rehabilitation

33. Documented signs and symptoms of a concussion in sports include all of the following, *except*:
    A. Amnesia (retrograde/antegrade)
    B. Loss of consciousness (LOC)
    c. Headache, dizziness, nausea
    D. Hallucination

34. The proposed mechanism of altitude/hypoxic training in sports like cycling include:
    A. Accelerated erythropoiesis as the primary hematologic effect
    B. Nonhematologic factors such as improved muscle efficiency at the mitochondrial level
    C. Glucose transport alterations
    D. Enhanced muscle-buffering capacity via pH regulation
    E. All of the above

35. Many sports injuries can be prevented if the athlete engages in an appropriate prehabilitation program to treat previous injury or to prevent future injuries using:
    A. Balance perturbation
    B. Plyometric training
    C. Stretching programs
    D. All of the above

33. D   34. E   35. D

CHAPTER 26

Diseases of the Muscle

1. Types of muscular dystrophy are the following, *except*:
   A. Duchenne
   B. Becker
   C. Emery Dreifuss
   D. Mc Ardles
2. Gower's sign is seen in:
   A. Duchenne muscular dystrophy
   B. Amyotropic lateral sclerosis
   C. Perthes' disease
   D. Hansen's disease
3. Stages in the rehabilitation of Duchenne muscular dystrophy are the following, *except*:
   A. Ambulatory stage
   B. Wheelchair dependent stage
   C. Stage of prolonged survival
   D. Stage of spasticity
4. Landouzy-Dejerine disease is also known as:
   A. Duchenne muscular dystrophy
   B. Limb girdle muscular dystrophy
   C. Facioscapulohumeral muscular dystrophy
   D. None of the above
5. The following is autosomal dominant:
   A. Duchenne muscular dystrophy
   B. Limb girdle muscular dystrophy Type 2A
   C. Facioscapulohumeral dystrophy
   D. Becker's muscular dystrophy

1. D   2. A   3. D   4. C   5. C

6. **CPK levels in Duchenne muscular dystrophy are:**
   A. Higher than the normal
   B. Only increased if the onset is in the second decade
   C. Directly linked to serum cholesterol levels
   D. All of the above
7. **Becker's muscular dystrophy is:**
   A. Autosomal dominant
   B. Autosomal recessive
   C. X-linked, absent dystrophin
   D. X-linked, reduced dystrophin
8. **Winging of scapula is usually seen in which of the following?**
   A. Becker's muscular dystrophy (BMD)
   B. Duchenne muscular dystrophy (DMD)
   C. Facioscapulohumeral dystrophy (FSHD)
   D. All of the above
9. **Inflammatory myopathy include all of the following, *except*:**
   A. Polymyositis
   B. Dermatomyositis
   C. Inclusion body myositis (IBM)
   D. Paramyotonia congenita
10. **Absent dystrophin or less than 3% of normal is diagnostic of:**
    A. Becker's muscular dystrophy
    B. Limb-girdle muscular dystrophy
    C. Duchenne's muscular dystrophy
    D. Facioscapulohumeral dystrophy
11. **Duchennes and Beckers muscular dystrophy mostly affects:**
    A. Girls and boys equally
    B. Adult women
    C. Girls
    D. Boys
12. **The most common form of childhood muscular dystrophy is:**
    A. Duchenne muscular dystrophy
    B. Limb-girdle muscular dystrophy
    C. Facioscapulohumeral dystrophy
    D. Becker's muscular dystrophy

6. A   7. D   8. C   9. D   10. C   11. D   12. A

Chapter 26: Diseases of the Muscle

13. **Which of these statements is true about Duchenne muscular dystrophy:**
    A. It affects predominantly young female children
    B. It can affect the cardiac muscle
    C. Afflicted children have a higher than normal IQ
    D. The weight of these children is normal or slightly below normal

14. **All the following drugs can cause myopathy, *except*:**
    A. Steroids
    B. Statins
    C. Folic acid
    D. Antimicrotubular agents

15. **The following are useful in the rehabilitation of DMD, *except*:**
    A. Stretching exercises
    B. Enzyme replacement
    C. Bracing
    D. Gait training

16. **Myotonia is a:**
    A. Spasm of the muscle
    B. Uncontrolled movement of the muscle
    C. Delayed relaxation of the muscle following a contraction
    D. Incoordination of a spastic muscle

17. **The most useful clinical criterion to distinguish Beckers muscular dystrophy from Duchenne's muscular dystrophy is:**
    A. Lower limb weakness
    B. Gower's sign
    C. Weakness of neck flexors
    D. Continued ability of the patient to walk into the late teenage years

18. **Complications of DMD:**
    A. Cardiomyopathy
    B. Respiratory infections
    C. Scoliosis
    D. All of the above

13. B   14. C   15. B   16. C   17. D   18. D

Section IV: Medical Conditions Needing Rehabilitation

19. Consumption of which of the following can cause myopathy:
    A. Zidovudine
    B. Cocaine
    C. Alcohol
    D. All of the above
20. The following pattern of muscle involvement is seen in DMD:
    A. Distal muscles more involved than proximal
    B. Proximal muscles more involved than distal
    C. Upper limbs affected more than lower limbs
    D. Only lower limbs are affected
21. Early clinical features of facioscapulohumeral dystrophy include all of the following, *except*:
    A. Protruding shoulder blade
    B. Inability to whistle
    C. Deltoid muscle weakness
    D. Inability to extend the wrist
22. Duchenne muscular dystrophy (DMD) may involve all of the following, *except*:
    A. Pulmonary system
    B. Intelligence quotient (IQ)
    C. Gastrointestinal (GI) system
    D. Epidermal dysplasia

19. D   20. B   21. C   22. D

CHAPTER 27

Spinal Cord Injury

1. What is the consequence of disuse of muscle from among the following?
   A. Increase in muscle fiber cross section area
   B. Atrophy
   C. Decrease in fatiguability
   D. Dystrophy
2. Correct positioning of quadriplegic in supine position is:
   A. Hips extended and slightly abducted, knees extended, ankles dorsiflexed and toes extended
   B. Hips extended adducted, knees extended, ankles plantar-flexed and toes flexed
   C. Hips extended and slightly abducted, knees slightly flexed, ankles dorsiflexed and toes extended
   D. Hips extended and slightly abducted, knees slightly flexed, ankles flexed and toes flexed
3. Type of bladder involvement in patients with spinal cord lesions above T10 –T11:
   A. Automatic bladder
   B. Autonomous bladder
   C. Uninhibited bladder
   D. None of the above
4. If there is trauma at the spinal cord involving S1 myotome, then which of the following muscles are affected?
   A. Abdominal B. Knee extensors
   C. Hip flexors D. Ankle plantar flexors

1. B   2. A   3. A   4. D

Section IV: Medical Conditions Needing Rehabilitation

5. A temporary loss or depression of all spinal reflex activity below the level of lesion occurs in:
   A. Stage of spinal shock B. Stage of total recovery
   C. Stage of spasticity   D. Stage of gait training
6. The paraplegic should do the following, *except*:
   A. Lift himself (using pushups) in the chair every 10 minutes
   B. Protect the limbs against excessive cold or heat
   C. Use a mirror for detection of abrasions, blisters on areas not visible directly
   D. Apply a hot water bottle over the suprapubic region whenever unable to micturate
7. The following finding is true about Brown-Séquard's syndrome:
   A. Ipsilateral motor loss and incomplete spinal cord injury
   B. Contralateral motor loss and incomplete spinal cord injury
   C. Ipsilateral motor loss and complete spinal cord injury
   D. Contralateral motor loss and complete spinal cord injury
8. At what neurological level of spinal cord injury is the patient at risk of developing autonomic dysreflexia?
   A. T4 and above   B. T6 and above
   C. T8 and above   D. T10 and above
9. A person with spinal cord injury develops signs and symptoms of autonomic dysreflexia. What should be done next?
   A. Bowel management
   B. Foley's catheterization
   C. Sit the person up and loosen any tight clothing
   D. Oral nifedipine
10. What is the classification of a pressure ulcer with full thickness skin loss involving subcutaneous tissue, muscle, bone and tendon?
    A. Stage I   B. Stage II
    C. Stage III   D. Stage IV
11. What are the long-term complications of an indwelling catheter in patients with spinal cord injury?
    A. Hydronephrosis   B. Kidney stones
    C. Pyelonephritis   D. All of the above

5. A   6. D   7. A   8. B   9. C   10. D   11. D

12. In the American Spinal Injury Association (ASIA) examination, the C6 myotome correlates with what muscle group?
    A. Elbow flexors
    B. Long finger flexors
    C. Elbow extensors
    D. Wrist extensors
13. In the American Spinal Injury Association (ASIA) examination, the umbilicus is the key dermatome for what level?
    A. T6
    B. T8
    C. T10
    D. L2
14. When no motor and sensory function is preserved in the sacral segments S4–5, it is called as:
    A. Complete spinal cord injury
    B. ASIA B
    C. ASIA C
    D. Incomplete spinal cord injury
15. Incomplete motor function is preserved below the neurological level, and less than half of the key muscles below the neurological level have a muscle grade less than 3. What is this ASIA grade:
    A. ASIA A
    B. ASIA B
    C. ASIA C
    D. ASIA D
16. The power of iliopsoas is used for testing which myotome:
    A. L1
    B. L2
    C. L3
    D. L4
17. Which of the following is true about detrusor sphincter dyssynergia:
    A. A common bladder condition seen in spinal cord injury patients
    B. It is the impaired coordination between detrusor and external urethral sphincter during voiding
    C. This increases the risk of high-voiding pressures and vesicoureteral reflux
    D. All of the above

12. D   13. C   14. A   15. C   16. B   17. D

Section IV: Medical Conditions Needing Rehabilitation

18. The following about heterotopic ossification is true:
    A. Formation of true bone in ectopic sites
    B. It can present with swelling, limited mobility, or pain
    C. It mostly occurs at the hips in spinal cord injury
    D. The risk is greater in complete spinal cord injuries, elderly and patients with spasticity and pressure ulcers
    E. All of the above
19. Which among the following is the leading cause of death in long-term paraplegics?
    A. Urinary tract infection (UTI)
    B. Heart disease
    C. Pressure ulcers
    D. Pneumonia
20. Which of the following statements is false? The spinal column consists of:
    A. Total 33 vertebrae
    B. 7 cervical vertebrae
    C. 10 thoracic vertebrae
    D. 5 lumbar vertebrae
21. Which statement about lateral corticospinal tracts is false?
    A. Ascending pathway in the spinal cord.
    B. Controls voluntary muscle activity
    C. 80-90% of the axons cross over to the contralateral side at the pyramidal decussation in the medulla
    D. 10-20% of axons that do not decussate travel in the ventral corticospinal tracts
22. Pain and temperature from the contralateral side of the body is transmitted by:
    A. Corticospinal tracts
    B. Spinothalamic tracts
    C. Spinocerebellar tracts
    D. Vestibulospinal tracts
23. The spinal cord receives blood supply from:
    A. 1 anterior and 1 posterior spinal arteries
    B. 2 anterior and 1 posterior spinal arteries
    C. 1 anterior and 2 posterior spinal arteries
    D. 2 anterior and 2 posterior spinal arteries

18. E   19. D   20. C   21. A   22. B   23. C

Chapter 27: Spinal Cord Injury

24. **All of the following are true about spinal cord tumors, *except*:**
    A. The most common primary tumors are glial in origin
    B. The majority of spinal cord tumors are metastatic in origin
    C. 95% of metastatic spinal cord tumors are intradural
    D. Approximately 70% of spinal metastasis occurs in the thoracic spine

25. **Which among the following is the most restrictive cervical orthosis?**
    A. Philadelphia collar
    B. SOMI brace
    C. Minerva brace
    D. Halo

26. **Jefferson fracture is:**
    A. C1 burst fracture
    B. C2 burst fracture
    C. T1 burst fracture
    D. T2 burst fracture

27. **Hangman fracture is:**
    A. C1 burst fracture
    B. C2 burst fracture
    C. T1 burst fracture
    D. T2 burst fracture

28. **All of the following about Chance fracture are true, *except*:**
    A. It is a transverse fracture of thoracic or lumbar spine from posterior to anterior through the spinous process, pedicles, and vertebral body
    B. Usually affects T12, L1, L2 levels
    C. Previously was most commonly seen in patients wearing lap seat belts. Now typically due to falls/crush injury with acute hyperflexion of the thorax
    D. Are so called because they are detected by chance on radiological screening

29. **All of the following are true about central cord syndrome, *except*:**
    A. Most common among incomplete SCI syndromes
    B. Produces no sacral sensory sparing
    C. Greater motor weakness in the upper limbs than the lower limbs
    D. More common in older patients

24. C   25. D   26. A   27. B   28. D   29. B

30. Orthostatic hypotension treatment includes all of the following, *except*:
    A. Repositioning
    B. Elastic stockings/abdominal binder
    C. Carotid sinus massage
    D. Mineralocorticoids

30. C

CHAPTER 28

Movement Disorders

1. Parkinsonism is one of the disorders of the extra-pyramidal system due to damage of:
   A. Basal ganglia
   B. Cerebral cortex
   C. Cerebellum
   D. None of the above
2. In Parkinsonism there is a deficiency of this chemical:
   A. Dopamine
   B. Histamine
   C. Dystrophin
   D. Adrenaline
3. Ataxia, dysarthria, nystagmus and intention tremor are caused due to damage of:
   A. Cerebrum
   B. Medulla oblongata
   C. Cerebellum
   D. Spinal cord
4. In Parkinsons disease, the following signs are present, *except*:
   A. Slowness of movements
   B. Cogwheel rigidity
   C. Macrographia
   D. Mask like facies
5. Nonstereotyped, unpredictable, jerky movements that interfere with purposeful motion:
   A. Athetosis
   B. Chorea
   C. Tics
   D. Dystonia
6. Difficulty in the placement of body part in space due to cerebellar lesions and lack of control of trajectory during active movement:
   A. Dystonia
   B. Asynergia
   C. Chorea
   D. Dysmetria

1. A   2. A   3. C   4. C   5. B   6. D

Section IV: Medical Conditions Needing Rehabilitation

7. The following statements about essential tremor are true, *except*:
   A. Tremor attenuates or vanishes with intake of small amounts of alcohol
   B. Tremors occur during movement or stress and less noticeable at rest
   C. It leads to medical complications in later life
   D. It is the most common type of tremor
8. Difficulty with quick, fine, alternating repetitive movement:
   A. Dysdiadochokinesis
   B. Dysmetria
   C. Dystonia
   D. None of the above
9. The most common type of focal dystonia is:
   A. Blepharospasm
   B. Cervical dystonia
   C. Generalized dystonia
   D. Autoimmune dystonia
10. Parkinsonism can be caused by all of the following, *except*:
    A. Mebendazole overdose
    B. Manganese toxicity
    C. Brain tumors
    D. Metoclopramide
11. 'Freezing' is a phenomenon in Parkinsonism where:
    A. The patient has frozen facial features
    B. The patient cannot tolerate cold climates
    C. The patient prefers a cold climate
    D. The patient finds it difficult to start or restart an activity
12. Cogwheel rigidity in Parkinson's disease is due to:
    A. Associated bradykinesia
    B. Tremor superimposed on rigidity
    C. Associated cerebellar lesions
    D. Fluctuating spasticity
13. The following are anticholinergic agents (muscarinic receptor antagonists) used in treating Parkinsonism, *except*:
    A. Trihexyphenidyl B. Benztropine
    C. Bromocriptine   D. Procyclidine

7. C   8. A   9. B   10. A   11. D   12. B   13. C

Chapter 28: Movement Disorders

14. Deep brain stimulation in the treatment of Parkinsonism involves the stimulation of all, *except*:
    A. Thalamus
    B. Hypothalamus
    C. Subthalamic nucleus
    D. Globus pallidus interna

15. The following are true about Parkinson plus syndromes, *except*:
    A. They usually get better with treatment as compared with Parkinsons disease
    B. Progressive supranuclear palsy is one of the common types
    C. Do not respond well to levodopa
    D. There are additional features of neurodegenerative lesions in Parkinson plus syndromes

16. The syndromes of multisystem atrophy (Parkinsonian type) are all, *except*:
    A. Shy-Drager syndrome
    B. Olivopontocerebellar atrophy
    C. Striatonigral degeneration
    D. Amyotropic lateral sclerosis

17. The classic features of Huntington's disease are all, *except*:
    A. Chorea/choreoathetosis
    B. Dementia and personality disorders
    C. Sex-linked recessive inheritance
    D. Family history (dominant inheritance)

18. One of these ataxias is not hereditary:
    A. Friedreich's ataxia (FA)
    B. Ataxia-telangiectasia (AT)
    C. Spinocerebellar ataxias
    D. Multiple system atrophy, cerebellar type

19. Specific interventions in cerebellar conditions may include the following, *except*:
    A. Effleurage
    B. Treadmill training
    C. Virtual game-based coordination exercises
    D. Visual-guided exercises for stepping

14. B   15. A   16. D   17. C   18. D   19. A

Section IV: Medical Conditions Needing Rehabilitation

20. **In restless legs syndrome:**
    A. The patients usually complain of pain in the upper extremities
    B. The cause is usually a surge in opioid levels in the brain
    C. Often associated with sleep and is worse with inactivity
    D. All of the above

21. **The following are useful in patients with Parkinson's disease, *except*:**
    A. Swivel fork and spoons
    B. Tone inhibiting KAFO
    C. Wheeled walkers
    D. Weighted utensils

22. **Nonpharmacologic measures used in multiple system atrophy (MSA) include which of the following:**
    A. Elevating the head of the bed and increasing salt and fluid intake
    B. Avoiding heat
    C. Fall prevention
    D. All of the above

23. **All of the following are true about levodopa-induced dyskinesias (LID), *except*:**
    A. Characterized by choreic movements of the extremities, trunk, and neck
    B. Eventually affects more than 40% of patients receiving sustained levodopa treatment for more than 6 years
    C. Management includes increasing the dose of levodopa
    D. A drug useful in such cases is amantadine

20. C   21. B   22. D   23. C

CHAPTER
29
Cardiopulmonary Rehabilitation

1. **ARDS stands for:**
   A. Acute renal distress syndrome
   B. Acute respiratory distress syndrome
   C. Acute radiating nerve symptoms
   D. Avascular retinal distress syndrome
2. **Postural hypotension is an abnormal fall in blood pressure of:**
   A. At least 20 mm Hg systolic and 10 mm Hg diastolic—within three minutes of standing upright
   B. At least 30 mm Hg systolic and 20 mm Hg diastolic—within three minutes of standing upright
   C. At least 40 mm Hg systolic and 10 mm Hg diastolic—within ten minutes of standing upright
   D. At least 30 mm Hg systolic and 20 mm Hg diastolic—within ten minutes of standing upright
3. **The primary muscle of respiration during inspiration is:**
   A. External intercostals
   B. Sternocleidomastoid
   C. Diaphragm
   D. Pectoralis major
4. **Accessory muscles of respiration are all of the following, *except*:**
   A. Sternocleidomastoid
   B. Trapezius
   C. Pectoralis minor
   D. External intercostals and scalene

1. B   2. A   3. C   4. C

Section IV: Medical Conditions Needing Rehabilitation

5. The greatest volume of air that can be exhaled from the lungs after maximum inspiration is called:
   A. Total lung capacity (TLC)
   B. Vital capacity (VC)
   C. Forced vital capacity (FVC)
   D. Functional residual capacity (FRC)
6. The amount of air within the lungs at the end of maximal inspiration:
   A. Total lung capacity (TLC)
   B. Vital capacity (VC)
   C. Forced vital capacity (FVC)
   D. Functional residual capacity (FRC)
7. The amount of air in the lungs at the end of maximal expiration:
   A. Vital capacity (VC)
   B. Forced vital capacity (FVC)
   C. Functional residual capacity (FRC)
   D. Residual volume (RV)
8. Causes of restrictive pulmonary disease include all of the following, *except*:
   A. Duchenne's muscular dystrophy (DMD)
   B. Amyotrophic lateral sclerosis (ALS)
   C. Chronic obstructive pulmonary disease (COPD)
   D. Guillain-Barré syndrome (GBS)
9. Nonpharmacologic prevention of exercise-induced bronchospasm includes all of the following, *except*:
   A. Warm up period for at least 10 minutes prior to exercise
   B. During cold weather cover the mouth and throat
   C. Avoid pollutants and aeroallergens
   D. Increase the intensity of exercise
10. Controlled breathing techniques to improve pulmonary function parameters include all of the following, *except*:
    A. Diaphragmatic breathing
    B. Segmental breathing
    C. Both of the above
    D. None of the above

5. B   6. A   7. D   8. C   9. D   10. C

Chapter 29: Cardiopulmonary Rehabilitation

11. Technique to reduce dyspnea and the work of breathing in the short term, from among the following:
    A. Pursed-lip breathing
    B. Huffing
    C. Mechanical insufflator-exsufflator
    D. Diaphragmatic breathing
12. Airway Secretion Management Program may include which of the following:
    A. Controlled cough and huffing
    B. Postural drainage
    C. Percussion and vibration
    D. All of the above
13. The most effective method of mechanical assistance for secretion clearance in a paralyzed patient is:
    A. Manually assisted cough
    B. Suctioning
    C. Mechanical insufflator-exsufflator
    D. Postural drainage
14. Management of obstructive sleep apnea include all of the following, *except*:
    A. Lose weight and quit smoking
    B. Sleeping pills
    C. Sleep on your side or abdomen rather than on your back
    D. Continuous positive airway pressure (CPAP)
15. Plastic tracheostomy tubes include all of the following, *except*:
    A. Shiley   B. Portex
    C. Jackson   D. Bivona
16. Which of the following statements about phases of cardiac rehabilitation is false:
    A. Phase I is during acute inpatient hospitalization
    B. Phase II is supervised outpatient cardiac rehabilitation lasting 3–6 months
    C. Phase III/IV (intermediate and maintenance periods): Maintenance phase in which physical fitness and risk factor reduction are accomplished in a minimally supervised or unsupervised setting
    D. Phase V is when the patient is fit to attend to his or her ADL's independently

11. A   12. D   13. C   14. B   15. C   16. D

Section IV: Medical Conditions Needing Rehabilitation

17. All of the following are true about metabolic equivalent (MET), *except*:
    A. Defined as the ratio of working metabolic rate to basal (resting) metabolic rate
    B. 1 MET = 3.5 mL O_2 consumed per kilogram of body weight per minute
    C. 1 MET = Energy consumption while at basal metabolic rate
    D. 1 MET is the measure of energy consumption by a normal individual per minute of moderate aerobic exercise.

18. Candidates for inpatient cardiac rehabilitation include all of the following, *except*:
    A. Patients who have had myocardial infarction
    B. Coronary artery bypass surgery (CABG) or angioplasty patients
    C. Heart failure and arrhythmias
    D. Unstable angina

19. Absolute contraindications for entry into inpatient and outpatient exercise training in cardiac rehabilitation include all of the following, *except*:
    A. Post-myocardial infarction
    B. Resting systolic blood pressure >200 mm Hg or resting diastolic blood pressure >110 mm Hg
    C. Moderate to severe aortic stenosis
    D. Acute systemic illness or fever

20. Target heart rate (THR) which is used to decide exercise intensity is calculated based on all of the following, *except*:
    A. Clearance heart rate method
    B. Age-predicted method
    C. Sex-predicted method
    D. Karvonen method

21. Physiologic response of the transplanted heart is different than the one seen in a post-CABG patient. All of the following statements are true about the transplanted heart, *except*:
    A. High resting heart rate due to parasympathetic denervation
    B. Lower peak exercise heart rate
    C. Resting hypertension is common, caused in part by the renal effects of antirejection medications
    D. Faster post-exercise return to resting heart rate

17. D   18. D   19. A   20. C   21. D

CHAPTER 30

Vascular and Hematological Conditions

1. In Volkmann's ischemic contracture there is flexion of all, *except*:
   A. Wrist
   B. Shoulder
   C. Fingers
   D. Hand
2. Classic hemophilia A is a blood coagulation disorder caused by:
   A. Factor IX deficiency
   B. Factor X deficiency
   C. Factor VIII deficiency
   D. Factor VII deficiency
3. Christmas disease is caused by deficiency of:
   A. Factor IX
   B. Factor X
   C. Factor VIII
   D. Factor VII
4. The cause of arthritis in hemophiliacs is due to the deposit of:
   A. Calcium hemoglobinate into the joint
   B. Hemosiderin into the synovial lining
   C. Crystal form of albumin and globulin from the blood into the joint
   D. Platelets in the exudate
5. The first line of care in hemophilic arthritis on observing a minor bleed into the joint are all, *except*:
   A. Immobilization
   B. Rest
   C. Icing
   D. Joint aspiration

1. B   2. C   3. A   4. B   5. D

Section IV: Medical Conditions Needing Rehabilitation

6. The ankle-brachial index (ABI) values are considered to be low-normal when:
   A. They are more than 1.0
   B. They are more than 1.5
   C. They are less than 1.0
   D. They are less than 0.5
7. The standard evaluation tool to establish lymphatic flow patterns is:
   A. Lymphoscintigraphy
   B. MRI scans
   C. CT scans
   D. Lymphangiography
8. Sickle cell disease can cause:
   A. Painful crisis   B. Osteonecrosis
   C. Dactylitis   D. All of the above
9. Intermittent claudication indicates:
   A. Poor lymphatic drainage of the lower limbs
   B. Possibility of TIA
   C. An inadequate supply of arterial blood to contracting muscles
   D. All of the above
10. Self-care measures in the rehabilitation of peripheral arterial disease include all, *except*:
    A. Extremes of temperature should be avoided
    B. The feet should be washed carefully with mild soap and warm water
    C. The patient is instructed to wear protective footwear at all times
    D. The patient should avoid any form of exercise
11. Which of the following is true about peripheral arterial disease (PAD):
    A. If the patient is active, intermittent claudication is the typical presenting complaint
    B. If the patient is inactive, then rest pain, ulceration, dependent rubor, or gangrene may be the presenting finding
    C. Patients with intermittent claudication have a significantly higher mortality than age-matched controls
    D. All are true

6. C   7. A   8. D   9. C   10. D   11. D

Chapter 30: Vascular and Hematological Conditions

12. Which of the following statements about ankle-brachial index (ABI) is false:
    A. The ABI provides objective data about arterial perfusion of the lower limbs
    B. ABI is a non-invasive test
    C. ABI values are considered to be abnormally low when less than or equal to 0.90
    D. The risk of death, usually from a cardiovascular event, increases dramatically as the ABI increases
13. In deep vein thrombosis, predisposing risk factors are all of the following, *except*:
    A. Hemophilia
    B. Prolonged immobilization during car or plane trips
    C. Use of estrogen
    D. Previous history of deep vein thrombosis or family history of thrombosis
14. The method of choice to investigate veins of the superficial, deep, and perforating systems:
    A. SpO$_2$ levels
    B. Ankle brachial index
    C. Duplex ultrasound
    D. X-rays of the lower limb
15. The following are true about thromboprophylaxis of venous system and the management of lymphatic disorders, *except*:
    A. Provision of knee-length compression stockings
    B. Graduated compression with decreasing pressure from distal to proximal is usually provided
    C. Compression pressure of 130–140 mm Hg (at the ankles)
    D. Limb elevation reduces edema
16. Paradoxical embolism occurs in deep vein thrombosis when:
    A. There is a defect in the heart, like a septal defect
    B. The embolus disappears on Doppler studies but causes symptoms
    C. The clot travels down through the veins of the leg
    D. The thrombus simultaneously forms in the deep arteries of the leg

12. D   13. A   14. C   15. C   16. A

Section IV: Medical Conditions Needing Rehabilitation

17. **Comprehensive treatment regimens for lymphedema include which of the following:**
    A. Skin care management and treatment of infection
    B. Specialized massage techniques to promote the movement of lymph
    C. Elevation and exercises to reduce swelling and supplement the massage
    D. All of the above

18. **All of the following are true about hemophilic arthropathy, *except*:**
    A. Hemophilia is a blood coagulation disorder caused by factor VIII deficiency (classic hemophilia A)
    B. X-linked dominant disorder, predominantly in females
    C. Elbow, knee and wrist are commonly involved
    D. Arthritis is caused by synovial proliferation and pannus formation

19. **Parahemophilia is due to lack of:**
    A. Factor IV
    B. Factor I
    C. Factor V
    D. Factor VII

17. D   18. B   19. C

CHAPTER 31

Arthritis

1. Bamboo spine is seen in:
   A. Rheumatoid arthritis
   B. Ankylosing spondylitis
   C. Reiter's syndrome
   D. Spinal muscular atrophy
2. Pauciarticular, polyarticular and systemic are types of:
   A. Osteoarthritis
   B. Juvenile rheumatoid arthritis
   C. Ankylosing spondylitis
   D. Gouty arthitis
3. The joint to be involved earliest in ankylosing spondylitis is:
   A. Spine
   B. Hips
   C. Sacroiliac joints
   D. Costochondral joints
4. Which is not a seronegative spondyloarthropathy?
   A. Ankylosing spondylitis
   B. Reiter's disease
   C. Rheumatoid arthritis
   D. Psoriatic arthritis
5. In Reiter's syndrome the classic triad is:
   A. Urethritis, arthritis, psoriasis
   B. Conjunctivitis, psoriasis, arthritis
   C. Arthritis, urethritis, uveitis
   D. Arthritis, urethritis, conjunctivitis

1. B   2. B   3. C   4. C   5. D

Section IV: Medical Conditions Needing Rehabilitation

6. **Tophi are seen in:**
   A. Rheumatoid arthritis
   B. Gout
   C. Ankylosing spondylitis
   D. Sjogrens syndrome
7. **Ankylosing spondylitis is diagnosed by the following findings, *except*:**
   A. Reduced chest expansion
   B. Schober's test
   C. Barlow's sign
   D. Occiput wall distance
8. **The following deformities are commonly seen in rheumatoid arthritis, *except*:**
   A. Swan neck deformity
   B. Boutonniere deformity
   C. Z thumb
   D. Claw hand
9. **One of the modifications of the environment used in rheumatoid arthritis is:**
   A. Theraband
   B. Finger goniometer
   C. Tap with long handle
   D. Motorised wheelchair
10. **One of the self-help aids used in ankylosing spondylitis is:**
    A. Theraband
    B. Finger goniometer
    C. Weighted cups
    D. Long handled reacher
11. **Home modifications for advanced rheumatoid arthritis includes all, *except*:**
    A. Built up handles for the doors
    B. Storage rack placement
    C. Long handle bath brush
    D. Design of cooking range
12. **The following is classified under degenerative arthritis:**
    A. Rheumatoid arthritis
    B. Osteoarthritis
    C. Ankylosing spondylitis
    D. Gout arthritis

6. B   7. C   8. D   9. C   10. D   11. C   12. B

Chapter 31: Arthritis

13. Detectable bony enlargements in the distal interphalangeal joints in osteoarthritis are known as:
    A. Heberden's nodes
    B. Bouchard's nodes
    C. Kienbock's nodes
    D. Kohler's nodes
14. The following is not an NSAID:
    A. Ibuprofen
    B. Indomethacin
    C. Paracetamol
    D. Naproxen
15. Splints to reduce ulnar deviation are usually given in:
    A. Ankylosing spondylitis
    B. Osteoporosis
    C. Osteoarthritis
    D. Rheumatoid arthritis
16. The following factors are included in the ACR/EULAR classification system for rheumatoid arthritis, *except*?
    A. Joint involvement
    B. Serology test results
    C. Acute-phase reactant test results
    D. Gender-based results
17. The following is true in systemic lupus erythematosus (SLE):
    A. Avascular necrosis is never seen
    B. Steroids should not be used to manage SLE
    C. Arthritis is very common in SLE
    D. Butterfly rash is typically seen over the chest
18. In pseudogout, the following crystals are deposited in the joints:
    A. Calcium pyrophosphate dihydrate
    B. Calcium phosphate trihydrate
    C. Calcium urophosphate
    D. Calcium pseudophosphate
19. Which are the joints of the body earliest and commonly affected in rheumatoid arthritis?
    A. Ankle
    B. Spine
    C. Hip
    D. Hands

13. A   14. C   15. D   16. D   17. C   18. A   19. D

Section IV: Medical Conditions Needing Rehabilitation

20. **In a patient with painful rheumatoid arthritis, the following exercises are generally performed:**
    A. Aerobic exercises
    B. Strengthening exercises
    C. Isometric exercises
    D. Isokinetic exercises

21. **The most commonly used radiographic classification system for osteoarthritis of the joint is the:**
    A. Massachusetts scale
    B. Brodie's system
    C. Kellgren-Lawrence system
    D. All of the above

22. **All of the following are associated with HLA-B27 (+) serology, *except*:**
    A. Ankylosing spondylitis
    B. Osteoarthritis
    C. Psoriatic arthritis
    D. Reiter's syndrome (reactive arthritis)

23. **Swan-neck deformity in rheumatoid arthritis is:**
    A. Hyperextension of PIP joint with hyperextension of the DIP joint
    B. Hyperextension of the PIP joint with flexion of the DIP joint
    C. Flexion of the PIP joint with flexion of the DIP joint
    D. Flexion of the PIP joint with hyperextension of the DIP joint

24. **In patients with rheumatoid arthritis, rehabilitation of the hand involves all of the following techniques, *except*:**
    A. Joint protection
    B. Work simplification instructions
    C. Splinting
    D. Heat modalities followed by active range of motion exercise
    E. Joint fusion surgeries

25. **Schober's test is used in which of the following conditions?**
    A. Ankylosing spondylitis (AS)
    B. Systemic lupus erythematosus
    C. Reiter's syndrome
    D. Dermatomyositis

20. C   21. C   22. B   23. B   24. E   25. A

26. Which is the most common cause of neuropathic arthropathy?
    A. Osteoarthritis
    B. Septic arthritis
    C. Systemic lupus
    D. Diabetes
27. Sjogrens syndrome consists of all of the following, *except*:
    A. Dry eyes
    B. Carotid involvement
    C. Dry mouth
    D. Lymphocytic sialoadenitis

26. D   27. B

EU GSPR Authorised Reprsentative
Logos Europe, 9 rue Nicolas Poussin
1700, La Rochelle, France
Phone: +33 (0) 6 67 93 73 78
E-mail: contact@logoseurope.eu

www.ingramcontent.com/pod-product-compliance
Ingram Content Group UK Ltd.
Pitfield, Milton Keynes, MK11 3LW, UK
UKHW021831140426
5217IPUK00021B/1388